How to Develop Resilience in Your Children

5 Strategies for Raising Children to Have GRIT

Daniel Alexander

© Copyright 2022 - All rights reserved.

The content contained within this book may not be reproduced, duplicated, or transmitted without direct written permission from the author or the publisher.

Under no circumstances will any blame or legal responsibility be held against the publisher, or author, for any damages, reparation, or monetary loss due to the information contained within this book, either directly or indirectly.

Legal Notice:

This book is copyright protected. It is only for personal use. You cannot amend, distribute, sell, use, quote, or paraphrase any part, or the content within this book, without the consent of the author or publisher.

Disclaimer Notice:

Please note the information contained within this document is for educational and entertainment purposes only. All effort has been executed to present accurate, up-to-date, reliable, complete information. No warranties of any kind are declared or implied. Readers acknowledge that the author is not engaged in the rendering of legal, financial, medical, or professional advice. The content within this book has been derived from various sources. Please consult a licensed professional before attempting any techniques outlined in this book.

By reading this document, the reader agrees that under no circumstances is the author responsible for any losses, direct or indirect, that are incurred as a result of the use of the information contained within this document, including, but not limited to, errors, omissions, or inaccuracies.

A free gift for our readers

7 Tips to develop a growth mindset which you can download by visiting our website www.danielalexanderbooks.com

Table of Contents

INTRODUCTION 1

CHAPTER 1: GRIT AND GROWTH MINDSET 7

WHAT IS GRIT AND A GROWTH MINDSET? 8
    Grit 8
    A Growth Mindset 9
    Growth Mindset vs. Fixed Mindset 10
WHY A GROWTH MINDSET MATTERS 11
    "Growth Despite Success." 12
GRIT AND A GROWTH MINDSET IN CHILDREN 13
    Teaching Grit 14
    Teaching a Growth Mindset 15
THE FIVE CHARACTERISTICS OF GRIT 17
    Courage 17
    Conscientiousness 18
    Perseverance 20
    Passion 21
    Resilience 22

CHAPTER 2: STRATEGY 1—PASSION 25

WHY PASSION? 26
PASSION AND GRIT 26
HELPING YOUR CHILD FIND PASSION 31
    Historical 32
    Sports 33
    Cultural 34
    Social 35
    Bonus Activity—Dream Big Evenings 35
    It Takes Time 36
BECOMING INVESTED IN YOUR CHILD'S PASSION 37

CHAPTER 3: STRATEGY 2—COURAGE 41

How You Can Develop Courage in Your Child 42
 Rules for Being Courageous.. 47
Overcoming Anxiety to Foster Courage 48
Courage, Accountability, and Responsibility 51
 How to Instill Accountability... 53

CHAPTER 4: STRATEGY 3—PERSEVERANCE 55

Why Children Need Perseverance... 55
Where Perseverance Matters 56
 School 57
 Social and Relationship... 58
 Sports and Physical Activities 59
How to Instill Perseverance in Kids................................... 60
Fostering Perseverance in Cautious Kids 62
 Pressure—Both Internal and External 63
 Helicopter Parenting.. 65
 Having Negative Associations and Experiences............... 66
 External Stressors 67
Combating Frustration 68

CHAPTER 5: STRATEGY 4—CONSCIENTIOUSNESS.................. 73

Why Kids Need Conscientiousness 74
 Natural Conscientiousness Versus Taught Conscientiousness... 74
Fostering Conscientiousness 76
 Time Management and Communication in Conscientiousness... 78
Conscientiousness and Creativity.. 80
 Encourage What-If Scenarios 82
 Find Creative Solutions to Mistakes................................. 83
 Build Upon Your Child's Interests..................................... 83
 Avoid Asking Your Child Closed-Ended Questions............. 84
 Spend Time With Your Child Throughout Their Creative Process... 85
 Schedule Creative Time 85
 Encourage Risk-Taking When it Comes to Creativity....... 86

CONTINUED CONSCIENTIOUSNESS 87
   Let Your Teen Know They Have the Power to Make Good Decisions 87
   Model Empathy and Kindness 88
   Trust Your Teen To Be Safe, But Be Aware 88
   Keep Them Safe From the Blue Light Trap 89
IF NOTHING ELSE, BE CONSCIENTIOUS 90

CHAPTER 6: STRATEGY 5—RESILIENCE 93

WHY KIDS NEED TO BE RESILIENT 94
HOW TO BUILD RESILIENCE IN YOUR CHILD 95
   Emotionally Connect With Your Child 96
   Your Child Needs to Know You Will Keep Them Safe When it Counts 97
   Stop Fixing Your Child's Problems 97
   Problem-Solving Skills Are Really Important 98
   Label Issues, Not Behaviors 99
   Teach Them Coping Skills 100
   Promote Positivity 101
   Take Your Kid Outside 102
   The 7 Cs of Resilience 102

CHAPTER 7: SUMMARIZING HOW TO DEVELOP GRIT AND RESILIENCE 109

RECAPPING A GROWTH MINDSET 111
   The Changes You Need to Make For Your Child 113
PASSIONATE, PURPOSEFUL KIDS 118

CHAPTER 8: DO YOU HAVE GRIT?—STRATEGIES TO BECOME A GRITTY PARENT 125

   Set Goals and Make Them SMART 126
   Rediscover Your Passion 127
   Reflect on Your Purpose 128
   Stop the Negative Self-Talk 129
   Surround Yourself With the Right People 129
SMART GOAL SETTING FOR PARENTS 130
   Decide What You Want to Achieve as a Parent 132
   Setting Those Goals 133

  Review and Reflect *135*
 S**TRENGTHENING** Y**OUR** R**ELATIONSHIP** W**ITH** Y**OUR** K**ID**.................. 136
  Say I Love You, But Show it Too *137*
  Tell Your Child You Love Them *137*
  Be Unshakable Regarding Consequences of Breaking Rules
  .... *138*
  Empathize With Your Child *138*
  Play With Your Child Often *139*
  Set Aside Uninterrupted Time *139*
  Eat Together *140*
  Put Rituals into Place With Your Children *141*
  Look for the Good *141*
 R**ESISTING THE** U**RGE TO** C**OMPETITIVELY** P**ARENT**.......................... 142

CONCLUSION 145

REFERENCES 151

Introduction

It soon became clear that doing one thing better and better might be more satisfying than staying an amateur at many different things. - Dr. Angela Lee Duckworth

For so many parents, raising children can be fraught with uncertainty. "How do I raise my child to be successful, compassionate, and kind, but resilient?" This is a common question and if you're a parent asking questions similar to this, you're certainly not alone. Some parents get it right; some raise adequate adults, and others get caught up in the fear of failing.

Let's face it, most of us want to know that our children are happy and healthy. We hope that these qualities will lead to them becoming successful, but the truth is that success depends on a lot of other factors.

Children are tricky. They need to be inspired to greatness, and success cannot be demanded of them. Instead, they need to be nurtured, inspired, guided, and reinforced to become the adults we hope they will become.

For so many of us parents and educators though, too much time is spent on ascertaining the best parenting strategies with very little time being spent on the actual work required to develop our children. Let's say you aspire to grow a beautiful, blood-red rose bush. You go out and purchase the seedling, and all of the nutrients and equipment needed, taking care to pick the best books on how to grow your little seedling into the majestic flowering bush you desire. Once home, you pop your seedling on the front porch, place all of the tools and accessories next to it, and get to reading. And you read, and read, and read, and strategize, and agonize about the perfect spot to plant your seedling, the perfect level of nutrients, sunlight, and water it will need. For weeks on end, you educate yourself on how to grow your seedling until eventually, when you are ready, you return to your seedling. Only, it is now a brown, withered stalk of what could have become something great.

This example sounds a bit bizarre, doesn't it? But the truth is that far too many parents are agonizing over what tools are needed to grow their children into magnificent adults that by the time they decide on the right strategy, their opportunity has passed.

As a parent and educator, I have spent many years learning how to inspire and nurture children to develop into their best possible selves and I can tell you with absolute certainty that not every strategy will work for every child. Don't believe me? Just ask parents of multiple children how different each and every one of their kids is.

So what is the point of reading this book if no one strategy works for every child?

Good strategies are meant to be malleable and adaptable, and the foundation of almost any successful strategy or goal in life is grit!

Think about it for a second—no person, regardless of how small or big they are, can ever succeed without perseverance, passion, and tenacity.

When children are infants and toddlers, their grit is exceptional. Through sheer determination your baby will go from being completely helpless to lifting and controlling their neck, to holding their own bottle, sitting, standing, feeding themselves, and walking.

What happens once your toddler pushes past these milestones though? What happens to this determination?

That's where you come in.

As parents, we want to protect our children from pain, frustration, and discomfort. So much so that we begin to chip away at their biologically programmed determination and will to learn and develop. We begin to shield our children from anything that can cause them pain, or worse, disturbs our peace. Let me ask you, how often have you interrupted your frustrated child in order to complete their task just so that you don't have to hear their frustration or because you don't want your child to be frustrated?

In doing this you are essentially teaching them that when they experience life's challenges someone will come along and save them from all of their frustrations, fears, and pain. And, as adults, we know this could not be further from the truth, so why do we keep teaching our children that they don't need to be resilient?

What we should be doing is teaching our children to cope with problems and to accept failure as a learning curve. And this is where the principles of grit come in.

I am not saying you need to be cold and heartless. Quite the contrary! Grit allows your child to experience all of the world safely. It shows them that overcoming obstacles and situations is something to be proud of, and instills in them a sense of capability to take on whatever the world throws at them.

When children learn resilience, they can overcome obstacles and can learn to problem-solve their way to achieving their goals. They learn to deal with disappointments in a way that is healthy and does not prevent them from achieving the goals they have set out for themselves.

And isn't it the goal of every parent to say that they achieved their own goal of raising a child who is thriving in life and not just surviving?

Through my personal experience as a parent and as a child educator I have written How to Develop Resilience in Your Children to help you to raise strong, independent children.

By reading this book, you will discover the five characteristics of grit and why your child needs them. These five characteristics will help your child to learn how to overcome their fear of failure—seeing failure as an opportunity to learn from their actions and mistakes.

These strategies and techniques were developed over time as I struggled with my own children and the anxiety they faced as they grew and matured. In taking a step back, and reflecting on why my children were not growing up to be confident in their abilities, I was forced to take stock of some of the mistakes I had made. And as you will come to find out in this book, mistakes when seen for what they are, are a powerful change-maker.

I will guide you and show you how you are overprotecting your child and how it is hindering their mental development so that you can begin to institute the right behaviors from both you and your children to ensure success in whatever your child decides to do in their future.

I will show you how to develop and cultivate a growth mindset in your child so that they begin to see their dreams as tangible goals that can be achieved, and how to motivate and inspire your children through the ups and downs of life.

By instituting the advice and actions in this book, you will be able to help your child navigate their intense feelings of fear and failure, how to overcome stress, peer pressure, and anxiety, building your child up to be a strong, capable person.

Remember that all the reading in the world will never grow your child into the thriving person you hope them to be. Like the little rose seedling, you will need to institute the actions within this book as you are reading them so that you and your child can learn and grow together to be the resilient people you deserve to be.

If you have enjoyed reading this book, please leave a review with your feedback.

Chapter 1:

Grit and Growth Mindset

"Our potential is one thing. What we do with it is quite another." - Dr. Angela Lee Duckworth

The term Grit was coined by psychologist and former educator, Angela Duckworth. In her April 2013 TED talk on the subject, Angela explained that "Grit is a passion and perseverance for very long-term goals. Grit is having stamina, sticking with your future, day in and day out, and not just for the week or month, but for years. It is the determination to work really hard to make your future a reality. And, it is living your life like it's a marathon, not a sprint (Duckworth et al., 2014)."

In addition, Duckworth asserts what many life coaches and psychologists have been saying for decades, that grit is built on the foundation of a growth mindset. When a person develops a growth mindset, their belief systems lie in their ability to learn outside of the realms of what they deem to be their natural talents. A growth mindset is not based on intelligence alone but on the ability of the brain to grow based on positive effort and the experience of learning.

What is Grit and a Growth Mindset?

Grit, as you now know, is the ability to push through life's challenges and obstacles, overcoming them to achieve your life's goals.

Grit and a growth mindset go hand-in-hand but they are distinctively different. This is because you can have a growth mindset without grit but you simply cannot have grit without a growth mindset.

Those who have developed a growth mindset, and who really live and breathe this mindset, may develop grit as a natural byproduct, but grit requires a person to not only become tenacious through life but to not move the goalposts when it comes to their life-long goals and dreams. Grit drives a person to work smarter and harder to succeed and when this is coupled with a growth mindset, the union results in a force that is unstoppable.

Grit

While grit is a combination of five characteristics which will be discussed further in this chapter, the basic definition of the word is tenacity. People with grit are passionate, tenacious, conscientious individuals who work with unwavering perseverance toward their goals. In addition, grit requires courage and a strength of character to weather life's storms.

Now some, but not all of the characteristics of grit are apparent in people with a growth mindset, and that is why the two states of being marry up so well together. A growth mindset, however, is a much broader definition and is a way of life.

A Growth Mindset

People who have a growth mindset have a strong belief that they can learn anything, even if these skills are outside of their natural talents and basic abilities. They understand that through work and dedication that natural talent only gives people a temporary step up and that even those with talent will never get better at what they are doing if they do not work to better those talents.

People who have learned and developed a growth mindset understand that anything can be accomplished if they embrace the process of learning rather than being fixated on the end result, and that mistakes and obstacles are only opportunities that have been presented to learn.

The concept of a growth mindset is the belief that a person's intelligence isn't set from birth but can be grown and increased over time through continued work and dedication.

The term growth mindset was first outlined in some detail by Carol Dweck PhD in her 2006 book *"Mindset: The New Psychology of Success."* When Carol Dweck began her research, the belief was that a person was either intelligent or not intelligent and this belief was the model of success at the time.

This school of thought simply believed that some people were more intelligent or naturally talented than others and that people who succeeded outside of this measure of intelligence were nothing more than a fluke of nature. Ultimately, the end all be all measure of success was a person's IQ, and how talented they were rather than how much they applied themselves to achieving success.

This meant that those with a higher IQ would be more successful than those with a lower IQ and the notion that a person could succeed outside of "IQ" through hard work was not something that was plausible.

Some people still believe this school of thought to be true, regardless of what science now shows. This school of thought is called a fixed mindset.

Growth Mindset vs. Fixed Mindset

People with a fixed mindset believe that they have all the knowledge and skill they will ever have with no way to improve or have a limited capacity to improve before they plateau on their skills and abilities. They believe they can not increase their IQ by more than a point or two.

A fixed mindset generally leads to a person not living up to their full potential. A fixed mindset also has been linked to lower self-esteem and high anxiety levels.

People with a growth mindset tend to be more successful in school and their chosen career paths. When things get complicated, a person with a growth mindset finds a way to overcome the difficulties rather than give up because things get too hard.

A growth mindset can help children and adults cope better with adversity. Those with a growth mindset tend to have high self-esteem because they believe that failure is not the end of the line. They are able to turn a failure into a teachable moment, and they don't get down on themselves if they are not successful on the first try.

Why a Growth Mindset Matters

According to HARAPPA, an online learning forum, people with a growth mindset continue to carry determination and discipline even after they find success or achieve their goals.

On the flip side, many people with a growth mindset also continue to work hard to achieve goals even if they are unsuccessful the first time. Sometimes the goals change, and success is found and nurtured despite setbacks or failure to achieve the original goals.

HARAPPA gives us an example of each scenario.

"Growth Despite Success."

Akshay Kumar is a Bollywood superstar. He is considered to be one of the greatest successes in India's movie industry. Even though he is successful, he continues to hone his craft and take on challenges in new films. He leads a very structured life with a regimented schedule to stay at the cutting edge of his craft. (Matthews,. et al. 2021)

"Growth Despite Failure."

Tina Khanna, known by her professional name Twinkle Khanna has not found as much success in Bollywood as many people expected. Both of her parents are big stars in the industry, and she has been in several movies but never found the acclaim that her parents enjoyed.

She has found success in other ways, however. She is an interior designer and has several books on the market.

She used the growth mindset to pivot to different career opportunities and find success. Her perseverance has paid off despite the setback she had in Bollywood. (Matthews,. et al. 2021)

Grit and a Growth Mindset in Children

In life, most people display moments of grit as well as moments in which they lack perseverance.

Children often learn from what their parents do and not from what they are told, and so many will learn that perseverance and grit are flashes in the pan that happen only occasionally.

This flash in the pan mentality, while beneficial in the moment, can cause issues with kids learning to avoid the "hard stuff" in life and only focus on the things they feel they want to achieve. And, because kids are learning through action, not words, when they see their parents and other influential adults in life give up on their dreams and goals, they begin to mimic this behavior. Conversely, when surrounded by grit, these children will become determined to achieve their own goals and success.

Limiting language and a lack of appropriately modeled behaviors is often the biggest killer of grit and determination in kids. Children who are subjected to language which squashes their determination, or limits their belief in themselves, will begin to develop a defeatist attitude.

Phrases like, "It is better to help my child because they **struggle** with mathematics," or "My child just **doesn't have the talent** for football," instill in them the notion that they are not talented or good enough to achieve their desired results.

More harsh, limiting language like "stupid, slow, bad," or "unruly," further ingrains in the child's mind what they believe the outside world believes them to be, creating inner conflict with their own self-belief.

It takes patience, kindness, inspiration, guidance, and modeling for a child to develop true grit. You cannot tell your child what is expected of them and hope that they will become resilient and successful in life.

Children need to believe, at their core, that they can achieve anything they set their mind to and are prepared to work diligently and conscientiously toward, and they need to know that there is no such thing as a bad child, only poor behavior.

Always remember that it takes a thousand "you're brilliants" to undo one "you're stupid," and you, yourself, are going to need to display resilience and grit in modeling the right behavior for the kids in your life.

Teaching Grit

According to Dr. Duckworth, grit is the result of passion and perseverance, and from a psychological perspective, it is the non-cognitive ability to apply passion and persistence through life. This passion and persistence, coupled with a strong drive to succeed, is what creates success.

Children can be taught grit through modeling behavior and through equipping them with the right set of tools to navigate life.

Teaching a Growth Mindset

Children in mainstream schools usually fall into the trap of a fixed mindset in which intelligence and natural talent are valued over diligence and hard work. For kids to learn a growth mindset they will need to understand that sometimes life comes with struggle and that obstacles are just part and parcel of our journey through life.

Because of this, it is critical to normalize struggle and help your child create a mindset that allows them to see that challenges are only opportunities to learn. Children will always react badly to fear, it's a natural, biological response, but when struggle is no longer feared, children can tackle tough tasks with optimism and a sense of normality.

A close second to normalizing struggle is to encourage your child to actively participate in their struggles, and that means taking a step back to allow your child to at least try to solve their own problems.

Kids need to understand that there is nothing that they will experience that is finite, and that that struggle will pass quickly through hard work and perseverance. It's normal for kids to say, "I can't do this," and as their parent, it is your responsibility to let them know that they cannot do it *yet*. When children know that difficult tasks and problems are overcomeable it drives neuronal growth, and a positive mindset as well as instilling a sense of independence in the child.

Finally, from as young as possible, children should be encouraged to set themselves goals and should be shown how to achieve these goals. And, because children learn more from what you do and not from what you say, modeling the right behavior for them is crucial. Parents shouldn't be afraid to admit when they have made mistakes in achieving their own goals and should model the proactive steps taken to correct these mistakes.

Even better, ask your child to cooperatively problem-solve issues you, or they, may be trying to overcome in achieving said goals, and praise their diligence in helping you to create a solution. Try to avoid praising your child's intelligence or natural talents and rather praise their persistence and perseverance in achieving their goals, regardless of how talented they are.

The Five Characteristics of Grit

Since Dr. Angela Duckworth's initial TED talk in April 2013, more research has been done to fine-tune grit and the process required to create individuals who possess this trait. There is a common consensus among researchers that shows that grit consists of five characteristics.

Let's take a look at these characteristics and what they mean for your child in depth.

The South African College for Applied Psychology lists the five characteristics of grit as courage, conscientiousness, perseverance, resilience, and passion.

Courage

Courage can be defined in many ways but a common misconception about courage is that it is the ability to act with the absence of fear. This couldn't be further from the truth though and courage is actually the ability to act *despite* fear.

One of the core values of the school where I teach is courage, in which we define the word as, *'doing what is hard so that we can do what is right.'*

Grit requires you to be courageous and to act appropriately despite your fear and uncertainty about the outcome.

Teaching your child to be courageous and to act within their purpose, values, and beliefs will ensure that they grow up to be adults who instinctively follow their own moral compass rather than following the crowd.

Conscientiousness

Most dictionary definitions describe conscientiousness as a well-organized person or state of being. Conscientiousness is also described as an orderly state in which lists or categories are created in order to arrange them into themed groups. But remember that conscientiousness as a person and in life can be quite different.

In terms of grit, conscientiousness is the ability to take on life with attention and awareness of others and the finer details that are often overlooked.

In a digital, fast-paced world, split attention and the fallacy of multitasking have become the norm, but the truth is no one can actually multitask—it's not physically possible.

People who display high levels of conscientiousness, however, display a level of order and calmness in the tasks they complete and this elevates them above those who believe they can multitask. Conscientious people have the desire to make sure the action they are currently engaged in is done properly. They do not believe in throwing things together or rushing to get things done. Instead, they plot out the correct amount of time required to complete the action properly and will work diligently through the steps required to get things done well.

I, myself, am a very conscientious person. I tend to pay attention to detail and work smart to complete my given tasks according to the steps set out for me.

Having said that, if you were to look at my desk it would be covered by piles of the many projects I am currently working on. To others, these piles were seen as disarray and a mess. But, let me tell you, when someone needs something from that "mess" I will always know where it is, at what stage in the process it is in, and how much time is still required for the task to be completed. I always know where, when, and how, because I work conscientiously.

This form of organization is more common than not, especially among children who sometimes organize things in a way that makes sense to them but not always to the adults around them.

Always remember, your child is a unique individual, and if they can tell you their where, when, and how, and they are working within their beliefs and morals, they are working conscientiously.

Perseverance

Perseverance and persistence are the abilities to muscle through adversity with a positive mindset. And, because grit requires your child to set and keep their long-term goals, perseverance and persistence are needed, especially when obstacles arise.

The ability to overcome difficulties is admirable, and for modern children, long-term goal setting is perhaps more important than ever before. For your child to develop perseverance they will need to be instilled with daily habits and practices that encourage and facilitate their goals.

It is important that you help your child to understand that life is fraught with obstacles, and let's face it, as adults we know that sometimes life can be just downright cruel. But, goals, while sometimes moveable, are still achievable, regardless of how many obstacles are placed in one's path.

Some of the most elite athletes have had their aspirations to win championships thwarted by injury and illness, and while recovery can be slow, they still achieve their goals in the future. Why? Because perseverance and grit drives them to come back from their obstacles and they find a way to ensure they achieve their long-term goals.

Perseverance means not giving up when things get tough, and a mindset that understands that by working smart, and putting your head down to weather the storm will get you through the most challenging parts of life.

Passion

Passion is most commonly associated with strong or powerful feelings of love or adoration, but passion extends beyond these feelings of love and adoration. Passion keeps people working toward their long-term goals. It is the "why" or the motivation behind them pushing through adversity, and it is the driving force that inspires a person to get up and do what needs to be done to achieve success.

Without passion, a person is working without purpose and the chance of goals being achieved will be very slim.

Passion is an integral part of having grit simply because a person isn't going to spend a lot of time and effort working toward a long-term goal if they just like to do something or they don't know why they are doing what they are doing.

For myself, passion is the driving force, not just in my personal life goals, but in my hobbies and my self-development. It is, however, important to differentiate between likes and passions. For example, I like to work on crossword puzzles, play card games, and read mystery novels, but I am passionate about writing and education.

So, I work hard to perfect my writing skills, read about the latest education strategies, and take a Professional Development course to improve my teaching skills and fill my spare time with doing crosswords and playing cards.

Resilience

Resilience is the ability to bounce back from difficulty. Without resilience, overcoming life obstacles to achieve your goals will be extremely challenging.

People who are resilient have the ability to look at life with a positive outlook and are not easily rattled when things don't go their way. In fact, resilient people will see adversity as an opportunity to learn and better themselves. They understand that no problem is without a solution, and they seek to find what part they played in the issue cropping up in the first place. Once these problem areas have been identified, they seek to rectify the issues, minimizing the risk of the same issue coming up again.

Resilience demands optimism and an ability to embrace life for its ups and downs. When a person embraces positivity and optimism, the byproduct is more robust mental health and mental toughness.

Those who are resilient understand that some things in life are simply beyond their control but that there is always a choice in how you handle these situations. Resilience is the admission that the only thing one can control is how they act and react to the situations they find themselves in.

Chapter 2:

Strategy 1—Passion

"Passion begins with intrinsically enjoying what you do." - Angela Duckworth

While passion is an emotion, it is also an action and the driving force behind a person's conviction and determination to succeed in achieving anything in life. The objective in life should always be to pursue our goals with an insatiable desire to succeed.

Passion is one of those emotions that can and should be acted on because without action, passion will never result in success. It is passion that fuels your desire for anything in life and it is passion that will keep you motivated through the tough times and the seemingly insurmountable obstacles.

Kids who are taught that they don't have to complete tasks they dislike, or that they believe they are not good at are doomed to live a life without passion, and let's face it, it is our love for—or our passion for—what we do that helps us get over the stages we don't necessarily like.

Why Passion?

Passion is the driving force and the desire you have to achieve anything in life, regardless of whether the outcome is good or bad. It is Richard Branson's 17-year journey to space, and Magic Johnson's return to the NBA.

Life without passion is a life without purpose, and when a person does not know or does not believe they have a purpose, they are rudderless in the storm of life. The secret to living a life in which infinite dreams are achievable is to live with passion and purpose, and what greater gift to give our kids than to guide them to work with passion and purpose to succeed.

Passion and Grit

Albert Einstein once famously said, "It's not that I'm so smart, it's just that I stay with problems longer," and while this is certainly true for gritty people, one component of this now famous saying is missing—passion.

You see, Albert Einstein was passionate about what he did, even if most of us modern-day laymen still don't have a full understanding of what exactly it was that he did do, we revere Einstein as a genius. But what set him apart from all other theoretical physicists of his time was his passion to solve the problems at hand.

As you now know, grit is a two-part equation and it demands both perseverance and passion to achieve long-term goals, and like Einstein's now famous $e=mc^2$, without passion, grit is not possible.

Psychologists and psychiatrists have long subscribed to the notion that the best predictor of future behavior is past behavior, and this makes instilling grit in our kids an invaluable skill. This is not to say that grit can't be acquired later, but why would you want to wait and make your child struggle in later years when you could proactively change their future right now?

Before I discovered grit I gave sole credit for my successes to my diligence and single-minded approach to completing tasks. I studied harder than most of my friends and my vision for my future was clear, but it wasn't until later in life that I realized that my perseverance alone wasn't what drove my success. I was passionate—about education, about teaching mindset, and about the creation of independent children and adults.

And all of this got me thinking, I don't think I ever had a time in my life where I had the typical, "I should" mindset. I always wanted to succeed because passion drove my long-term goal. This is not to say that my own children didn't suffer from anxiety, and negative emotions in dealing with life's challenges but this journey to grit within our family was exactly that—a journey.

Before I realized that grit was a two-part equation, I only valued persistence, but all the grittiness in the world isn't going to help if you don't know why you are working toward your goals.

Without passion, your child will be led by fear, and success is never achieved through fearful action, but rather through a *love* of what you are doing. Think about it, if you fear heights, it's going to take a whole lot more energy to will yourself to take the next step on a high-up swinging bridge. But, if you change your mindset from fear to a love of conquering challenges, or an appreciation for adventure, the next step is justified without having to will yourself.

Is the fear still there? Sure! But the love for what is on the other side of that swinging bridge is far greater than the fear of remaining rooted in place or turning back.

And this is where mindset comes in because passion is the self-driving force behind success. It's never about what other people expect of you, and this means you need to create confident kids who are capable of articulating and acting upon their own expectations of themselves.

Fostering passionless persistence in your child is not grit. It is demanding perfection and it is absent of one intrinsic force: the self-motivation to succeed. Passionless persistence is the ability to take enough steps across that swinging bridge only to be overrun with fear and choosing to turn back halfway. Logically, turning back makes no sense. After all, it is the same amount of steps to the other side than it is to get back to what you know is safe, and a safety net is what non-motivated people crave when they face fear head-on.

To foster true grit in your kids you need to have a solid strategy in place that has passion steering perseverance.

To do this, you need to first learn about your child's passion and then fuel that passion. And this means letting go of what you want your child to be or achieve in life. You cannot live vicariously through your children—they have their life to live and you have yours. Since you are still living and fostering grit, it is time to do the same in your life and pursue your goals in the same way you hope they will pursue theirs.

Your only job when uncovering passion is to support your child. That's right. It really is that simple. Support their passions. Kids need to be exposed to a great many things for them to find what it is that ignites passion in them, and you need to be willing to support your child as they work through all of the things that spark curiosity in them. Some kids will try one or two activities and find their passion quickly, while others may go through a list longer than you can count.

Don't get me wrong, I am not encouraging a lack of commitment, on the contrary, it's just that some kids take longer than others to find what it is that sets their soul on fire, and I promise you, that's normal.

Grit encourages curiosity and attentiveness to what it is your kid keeps coming back to, and then peel back the layers of their favored activities to uncover their purpose. The easiest way to do this is to notice what makes your child feel like they are free of the pressures of life.

There is a method behind this madness; kids who are allowed to be curious, and who can explore everything outside of what they deem to be their natural talents, are more likely to tolerate the discomfort of being outside of their comfort zone.

When we raise children to believe that they are only great at things within their comfort zone, they never grow and they become intolerant of disappointment, pain, and failure. And here is the irony in staying within your comfort zone—it becomes extremely uncomfortable because human beings are meant to grow, both physically and mentally.

We are not designed to remain stagnant, and encouraging stagnation develops a feeling of being unsafe in a world that your child inherently knows is already not a particularly safe place. Teaching your child that it is great to pursue their passions gives them the courage to try things that are new, and in trying things that are new, they are overcoming fear, reframing it as excitement.

I don't know if you have watched the movie *The Croods*, and if you haven't you really should. The lead protagonist of the movie is terrified of anything new.

His daughter, the ever-curious Eep, is fueled by her passion for anything new that can lead her and her family out of the dull, problem-riddled life they are living. Eep guides her family, at first with baby steps, into the newness, until catastrophic events force her begrudging father into a new, uncomfortable, yet fruitful existence.

The reason I bring this film up specifically is because the catalyst for Grug's eventual leap into a new life is his love, and his *passion* for his family. The point that I am trying to make is that without this love, the Croods would have probably remained where they were, swallowed by the abyss of the changing world around them.

The same is true for your child. Guide and motivate their persistence with passion, not fear, and your kid will choose the right path more often than not, even if that path is a difficult one to travel, because it is passion that fuels their persistence.

Helping Your Child Find Passion

You may be wondering how exactly you can help your child find passion.

The answer is pretty simple but will require some work on your part.

Exposure to a variety of activities is a great place to start, but it is important to narrow these activities down so that your job of helping them to find their passion is a lot easier.

Asking your child outright what they are passionate about is likely to yield some interesting results that will probably vary from YouTubing to gaming, but these are not passions per sé and are more than likely avoidance behaviors your child is using to try and avoid what is happening in their lives or the lack of direction they have in their lives.

I have found that the easiest way to expose your child to a wide variety of activities that will help them to find their passion is to categorize these activities into historical, sports, cultural, and social activities.

Historical

Historical activities involve you exposing your children to activities and stimuli that incorporates history. This doesn't mean plopping them in front of the History Channel and hoping for the best, although some exposure to series and programs on history won't hurt. Cast your net wide with history activities and include sightseeing tours like trips to museums and libraries as well as offering reading materials and online resources.

Remember that history encompasses a great many subjects—not just wars and land discovery—and includes music, politics, the arts, science, and invention.

Allow your child to look at history for what it was and let them form their own opinions on the events that took place. Don't interfere with their opinions, no matter how hard that may be.

Sports

From early in your child's life they should be exposed to sports as it is a great way for them to develop hand-eye coordination and helps them to fine-tune both their gross and fine motor skills. Again, this is not having your kid sitting in front of the tv with you on a Saturday watching your favorite sports team, although this is a great bonding exercise.

Let them choose what sporting activity they would like to participate in, don't get involved, and then encourage them if they show passion, regardless of whether they are what you deem to be good or bad at the sport. Attend practices and matches, and allow your child a safe space to vent any frustrations they may have with the sport.

If your child is under the age of ten and is a little indecisive as to what sport they would like to participate in, feel free to offer guidance. The point is to encourage independence within expected boundaries.

Set a time limit for your child if they tell you they don't like the sport, asking them to reevaluate after a month whether or not they still feel the same way. Understand that your child may suddenly not enjoy their favorite sport because they feel they are not good enough, or they may be experiencing fear and it's your job to help guide them in navigating these feelings.

If, however, your child really just doesn't like the sport they have chosen, allow them to move on, no matter how frustrating their changing mind may be.

Imagine if Tiger Woods' mother denied him the opportunity to play golf because he wouldn't commit to tennis!

Cultural

Exposure to other cultures and languages is a powerful motivator in finding passion and it's pretty easy to incorporate into your child's life without much money or inconvenience involved. Speak with your spouse, or take initiative and institute cultural months in your home in which you immerse yourself in another culture. Learn the basics of the language from the culture that has been chosen, and help them to research the history, foods, and arts of that culture. Go to local events or suburbs that are historically cultural or arrange field trips in which your child can have a one on one experience with another culture.

Exposing children to other cultures develops general knowledge, encourages creativity and imagination, and helps to develop a broader awareness of the world around them. Getting your child involved in cultural activities can widen your net when helping them find their passion as culture involves everything from art and music to language, sports, history, politics, etc.

Social

Enrolling your child in social activities, specifically, those that incorporate service to others, is a great way to ignite passion as well as instill empathy in your child. Social activities are also a great way to spend time as a family while giving back to your community.

Volunteering as a family to work at local homeless shelters, animal shelters shows your child that they can make a difference in their community and in the lives of others with acts of service.

The point is not to make your child feel bad about what they have, rather it is to instill humility, and to show them that serving people can build a sense of community and an awareness of what is happening around them and that in taking action they can make a difference in another person's life.

Bonus Activity—Dream Big Evenings

Children will express their passions as far-fetched aspirations and big dreams. From astronauts to prima ballerinas and superheroes, these big dreams often cover up their true passion.

Kids who want to be superheroes may have a desire to be a leader or to help other people, and astronauts may have the desire to live a life of adventure. Children need to have their dreams and desires heard and encouraged, knowing that their parents value their big dreams.

Having dreams is as important as being realistic in our goals for our lives. Having evenings in which you let your child express their big dreams, and allow them to elaborate on their dreams will help foster passion.

It's never too late to start allowing your child to dream big, and in actuality, it's never too late for you to dream big too.

Allowing your child to dream big ensures that when they reach their teens they are less likely to experience self-limiting beliefs. And, as parents, allowing your kids to express their dreams gives the perfect opportunity to open up discussions about activities your child could do to encourage their passion to ignite.

It Takes Time

Finding passion isn't instantaneous, it takes time and a deeper sense of knowing one's self. Helping your child to find their passion is a step-by-step process, and it will take some time which is why it's important to allow your child to be curious and to explore in life.

You need to take time to develop an understanding of how your child's mind works, and in the process you need to encourage their efforts, not their intelligence and talents. You're going to need to work on this every single day and be understanding of the fact that as your child grows and matures, their passions may change.

It's the underlying purpose that drives the passion that will never change. Help your child to create a vision for their life and their future and reassure them that their life is malleable and will evolve as they do.

Helping your child to find their purpose will be their compass, pointing their passion in the right direction from a personal and professional point of view. Have your child make lists of the things they love in life so that they can begin to truly know who they are and what they believe their purpose is in life.

Becoming Invested in Your Child's Passion

Once your child has found what ignites their passion it's time for you to change gears and be the fuel that fans the flames of their fire.

First and foremost, don't push your child too hard. I get it, it's really easy to go into full cheerleader mode, pushing your child to excel in every single moment of their lives but do you know what happens when you fan flames in the wrong direction? They turn around and eventually burn out.

The point is to let your child work at their own pace, with diligence. Remember to allow them to create a slow, consistent burn. I mean, would you rather have a campfire that burns hot for 10 minutes or one that can keep you warm all night long?

If your child shares the same interests as you or is passionate about the same interest, try to allow them to grow and develop in the direction they choose. Just because you were an amazing writer who never had the confidence to write the next bestseller doesn't mean your writer child needs to fulfill your dreams of writing. Maybe your child's passion for writing will lead them down a different path from what your dreams and aspirations are, perhaps they will become a literature professor or the editor-in-chief for an international magazine. Allow your child to grow, develop, and evolve in the direction that suits them best.

Always remember that grit and a growth mindset go hand-in-hand and this means praising your child's efforts as well as praising their successes. Let your kid know that learning a new skill takes time and that there is no such thing as perfection. The greatest athletes in the world will try to improve on their techniques, even when they have reached their achievements.

Help them to steer their interests in a way that is organic and let them know that it's okay to fail, as failure is merely an opportunity to learn. Allow your child to express their fear and then encourage them to reframe their fear to excitement so that they can learn to step outside of their comfort zone and grow.

Passion, by nature, grows and evolves with a person. Grant your kid the freedom to develop in their passion and permit them to find their path in life. Don't distract them from new interests just because your child has found their passion.. Support and encourage diversity in their knowledge and their achievements.

Chapter 3:

Strategy 2—Courage

"Success is never final; failure is never fatal. It's courage that counts." — Angela Duckworth

Second to passion is courage. As explained earlier, courage doesn't refer merely to physical bravery. When it comes to your child, you need to remember that courage is never the absence of fear but acting despite of fear.

Instilling courage in your child will make sure that they stand up for what they believe in, even if that means standing alone.

When we examine courageous people a few qualities stand out:

Patience

Self-confidence

Conviction in their beliefs

Integrity

Leadership

Objectivity

Compassion

The ability to take action

Children need courage in order for them to try new things and to grow and develop in life—riding a bike, making new friends, going to school, etc. It helps them to do the right thing even when others are not. Courage also helps your child to admit to their mistakes and instills humility in them.

Without courage, it is difficult for your child to persevere through life's goals and challenges, and more importantly, without courage your child's self-esteem will not develop.

How You Can Develop Courage in Your Child

Everyone wants to feel safe. It is a basic need, but realistically speaking, no one goes through life without at least some scrapes and bruises. Let's face it, we all want our children to live a life in which they feel safe at all times but you cannot enrich your child, nor can you teach them about life's pitfalls by never letting go of their hand.

Nurturing bravery and courage in your child isn't about throwing them in the deep end, it's about taking them through the steps that develop courage as one of their core strengths.

Speak courage into them—Children will either step away from what is expected of them or they will step up to these expectations. Read that again! Your child will either flee life or they will face it head on and the only way for them to do this is for you to clearly define what is right and what is wrong and by speaking courage into them. Let them know that it's okay to not feel very brave in the moment but that action is the only way to move forward in life.

Let them know that there is no such thing as imperfection—Failure and rejection are part of life. We as adults know that and we understand that it can be tough on our self-esteem. You will need to let your child know that nothing in life is perfect and that every new experience they have will provide them with new information and new wisdom that will serve them in life. Allow your children to be imperfect and help them to see their ability to grow in their mistakes.

They'll never be ready and that's okay—From the moment people are born they learn to become comfortable. Comfort on their mother's chest, comfort in their father's arms, and comfort from their teachers as they enter into the education system. But, growth never comes from remaining comfortable. Any decision outside of what is comfortable is going to feel uncertain. Let your child know that they will never feel like there is a right time to change, and that courage means reframing fear as excitement. Teach your child to look at change as something that may feel uncomfortable but is exciting because they will grow from the new experience.

Introduce them to newness as young as possible—Routine is great but new experiences are just as important. Introducing your child to new concepts, creative outlets, experiences, feelings, smells, tastes, etc instills courage and confidence. And, when a child is exposed to newness from a young age, they are more tolerant of it as they grow. Show your child that it is okay to test the boundaries of what they believe are their mental and physical capabilities, and show them that they are not as fragile as they believe themselves to be.

Always model the behavior you want to see—If you want your child to be brave and courageous you need to show them what it means to embrace those attributes. Don't be indecisive around them, and definitely don't contradict what you have told them. This means not saying yes when you mean no and not people-pleasing to keep the peace. Be open with your child about your fears and how you overcame them but do not embellish on the truth. The point is to help your child see that humans overcome fear every day rather than building yourself up to be a superhero in their eyes. Your child needs to be able to see you as fallible rather than someone who has always known how to be brave.

Encourage them to vocalize their courage—It's really easy for adults, especially when they are busy, to listen with half an ear or to dismiss what our kids are saying. But very few kids are equipped with a verbal filter and they will more often than not speak to you about their brave acts before they actually go ahead and do something. By allowing your child to vocalize their courage you are teaching them that it is okay to stand up for what they believe in and to act on that belief. And, when your child practices their vocal courage it will feel less awkward when they need to push back against a friend, or someone they love or respect. I am not encouraging you to allow your child to be disrespectful, but with the right guidance, children can learn to question those in authority or those they respect in a way that is thought-provoking and encourages open discussion. Ask your child what their opinions are on certain topics and let them problem-solve some of the minor issues you may be facing in your life, and above everything, let them know that it's okay to have differing opinions.

Teach them the difference between action and reaction—Your child needs to know that there is a difference between them taking action and reacting to a situation. Courage requires a person to take action, not react on their emotions. You can gently guide your child by telling them that you love how passionate they are about life and then let them know that there are different ways to take action.

Encourage discussions about their intuition—Kids need to understand that intuition should be taken seriously and is not some hocus pocus magic. They should trust their gut instinct to do the right thing. Ask your child to describe how they felt in their belly and body when they decided to act courageously. Translate these feelings for them, highlighting them as excitement, not fear. But, be sure to tell them not to downplay their fear, especially in situations in which they are participating in risky behavior, or in which they believe the action is wrong.

Discuss self-talk all the time—Kids have a wonderful ability to talk themselves into and out of situations. Use this ability to your advantage by encouraging positive, encouraging self-talk. Children who have a positive internal dialogue will gravitate toward making the right decision in the moment and are less likely to follow what others are doing. Ask your child what is happening in their mind, explaining to them that an internal dialogue is a normal, human experience. Once your child understands that self-talk is normal, you can begin to help them develop their internal dialogue into one that is positive, uplifting, and morally correct. This will assist in eliminating self-limiting language.

Always encourage their sense of adventure—Kids are naturally curious and have a deep sense of adventure. Developing and nurturing your child's sense of adventure will have them being brave before their mind ever tells them they cannot do something. A sense of adventure can be anything from trying a new food or trying out new equipment on the playground. Whatever it may be, it's vitally important that you allow your child to explore, play, and tap into their natural courage.

Adventure helps your kid to discover what their current limitations are, and with a good sense of positive self-talk, your child will challenge these limitations.

Rules for Being Courageous

Sometimes being brave means doing things that push our limits, and sometimes being brave means doing the right thing. But kids often don't know or understand what the right thing is, especially when they are younger and are still trying to navigate the world around them. Rules, guidelines, motivations—whatever you want to call them—will have your child thinking before they act or react. Saying no to something that doesn't feel right, or goes against the values you have instilled in your child, will be one of the most courageous, and most difficult things your child will ever have to do. Giving your child a set of guidelines will make saying no a little bit easier, and will give them a little nudge in the right direction.

When your kid encounters a situation where they are unsure of what their intuition is telling them, let them run through these three questions:

Will my actions break a rule, or break the law?

Will my actions emotionally or physically hurt someone?

Does this feel right for me to do?

If your child answers yes to any of these questions they should not engage in the activity and should say no to anyone who is trying to influence them. Help your child commit these questions to memory, and let them know the importance of the guidelines put in place.

You want your children to display courage, not reckless abandon, and when they have a clear, concise tool to guide them it makes it easier not only for them to make a decision but for you to hold them accountable to their decision.

Overcoming Anxiety to Foster Courage

Parenting an anxious child can be a tough task, especially when it comes to fostering courage in a child that suffers from high levels of anxiety.

All kids are courageous to a certain extent but some kids are inherently more courageous than others. The good news is that courage is a teachable skill, and children who are more anxious naturally can definitely learn to be courageous.

The key to empowering anxious children is to allow the process of overcoming fear to be the reward and to push them outside of their comfort zone little by little. Your anxious child needs to understand that being courageous is about making the right choices first and foremost. And, when your anxious child freezes or chooses to run away from their fear, it's up to you to acknowledge their fear but also help them to see that they have a choice to overcome their fear.

Let's look at some ways that you can help your anxious child develop and nurture their adventurous, curious, and courageous side.

Plan activities that push your child outside their comfort zone—Start small with a child who is anxious. If your child is scared of bugs, taking them into a Fear Factor style challenge in which bugs are thrown all over them is just going to be counterintuitive. Kids who are afraid of bugs and other slithering or creepy crawly creatures can be introduced through a glass pane in a safe, educating environment. If they're afraid of swimming, introduce them to the water slowly, with floaters at first, and then without the floaters in a wading pool. It is important to let your child explore their limits within the confines of what they feel is safe before taking them one more step outside of their comfort zone.

Don't throw your child in the deep end—Children, even courageous ones, do better when they are educated about what safety measures are in place. You will need to let your anxious child know that the entire point of them taking on tasks that make them scared is to help them overcome their fear in a way that is safe and structured. Take them through any safety rules they may need to follow and highlight the positives of the experience at hand. When your child starts showing signs of fear taking over, remind them that they are safe and that you would never put them in danger.

Encourage mistakes—Anxious children need to know that making mistakes is a normal human process. When your child tries, but makes mistakes, praise them for their efforts and for the courage they displayed in trying in the first place. Never make a big deal of their failure. Rather, encourage your child to try again with the knowledge they have learned.

Don't downplay their feelings—Downplaying your child's feelings makes them feel unsafe, they need to know that their feelings and emotions are valid. Ask your child how they feel when they begin to meltdown or have made a mistake, or once they have completed the task at hand. Often children mistake excitement or feelings of intense joy for fear and it's important that you are on hand to acknowledge how they feel and help them to identify and reframe these feelings.

Don't forget to ask them about their process—Asking your anxious child what their process was when tackling a scary task gives you the ideal opportunity to praise their efforts in overcoming their fears. Ask questions like, "How did you feel when doing this? Would you change anything? Did you make any choices while you were doing the task?" If your child shows signs of hesitation or self-doubt, remind them of how far they came to do the task and let them know that they should be really proud of their efforts.

Don't discredit deep breathing—Sometimes your child will go from great to full fight or flight mode without warning. In moments like this, it is important that you don't panic, and that you don't take full responsibility for bringing your child out of their current mental state. Hand them the power by guiding them through deep breathing exercises or a mental distraction activity like The Five Senses Grounding Technique. Have your child breathe in time with you, focusing on your breath before letting them know they are now in control and that you will follow their breathing patterns. Once your child comes through the other side of their fear, have them affirm that they are always in control of what happens in their mind and with their body.

Courage, Accountability, and Responsibility

Adults, for the most part, understand what it means to be accountable and responsible for their actions, but children need to be taught that being these things takes courage.

Kids feel that being responsible or accountable means they are to blame for everything that goes right or wrong. Accountability can be explained really easily to children, especially when parents or the child's caregivers change their own mindset from one of a fixed outcome to a growth outcome.

Being accountable is simply being willing and able to share how an outcome came about. In other words what actions were taken, or not taken, and what thought processes went into creating the outcome at hand. Accountability is never about the result of the actions, or lack thereof. Rather allow your child to unpack their processes without fear of repercussion so that they can identify where they went wrong, and how they can improve in the future.

Accountability requires a person to not just be honest, but to work hard, and to do everything to the best of their ability so that they can act responsibly and share the information they have gathered while doing so. Your child should never be encouraged to be recklessly courageous, as this kind of courage often leads to the exact opposite of the desired result.

Courage without accountability and responsibility comes at any cost, and the damage caused from these actions is against the principles of the true purpose of courage.

As adults, we need to move away from the assumption that accountability lays the blame for anything that goes wrong on the person who is courageous enough to speak up and do the right thing. Instead, fostering accountable courage will develop future independent, kind, and strong individuals who make good decisions and who stand by their decisions.

How to Instill Accountability

Accountability begins with setting clear limits on what is permitted and what is not. Setting these boundaries ensures that your child knows what the rules are and sets them up for later life when there will be rules and laws to follow.

These boundaries should revolve around moral and values-based guidelines without limiting your child's creativity, curiosity, or courage.

For example, do not prevent your child from taking on rock climbing but give them a clear, concise set of guidelines as to what you expect of them when displaying the courage it takes to learn this new skill.

"I think it's fantastic you want to go rock climbing. I am here to support you completely! Please can you make sure that you follow all of the safety protocols that the climbing club puts in place? No climbing by yourself, no free climbing without the right safety gear, and no risky behavior. I know that you are a responsible person and you will make sure that your safety comes first."

Make sure that your kid understands the boundaries, and if they try to shift focus to someone else's actions, bring the conversation straight back to them being accountable for their own actions.

But, it isn't as simple as telling your child what they should not do. They need to figure out how to stay within the boundaries themselves and this is where listening to what your child has to say will come in handy.

"I hear that you're pushing back a little bit. Let's discuss how I can support your goals while still staying within the boundaries," or simply "How can I help you to stay within the boundaries I have set out for you?"

It's not your responsibility as a parent to ascertain whether or not your child thinks you are being fair. What is your responsibility is to ensure that your child is accountable for their actions and that they know the consequences of their actions.

This doesn't mean threatening with punishments as consequences, but it does mean that your child understands that every action they take can have a positive or a negative outcome and that since they are responsible for their actions, they are also responsible for the outcome.

Chapter 4:
Strategy 3—Perseverance

"The highly accomplished were paragons of perseverance."— Angela Duckworth

Perseverance is the ability to push through obstacles and hardships in life. Kids who are raised with perseverance are more likely to live a happy, balanced life because they are automatically instilled with a sense of pride.

When perseverance is coupled with courage, children feel that they can take on life, even if it is filled with challenges along the way. It is perseverance that will drive your child to move through the things that are difficult for them so that they can enjoy the things they like.

Why Children Need Perseverance

Kids need to be taught to persevere because life is tough at times, and as much as we would like to protect our children, at some point they are going to grow up and are going to need to push through, despite their discomfort.

Adults tend to think of perseverance as something that only applies to mental hurdles, but the reality is that perseverance encompasses anything and everything that is difficult. This can mean obstacles like learning a new physical skill, forming new habits, education, creative skills like arts and dance, and even social and relationship skills.

Children need to be taught that the hard task at hand doesn't matter as much as the perseverance and drive to push through—even when that task seems impossible. Without perseverance, no one would ever reach their goals, nor would they ever know how good it feels to succeed at the things that matter to them.

Kids need to be taught that there is no easy way to get through struggles and challenges, and when they quit or avoid challenging situations, the issue doesn't go away. Often, the issue at hand will become harder and more challenging, requiring more perseverance and grit to get through it.

Where Perseverance Matters

Kids will be confronted with a different set of circumstances where perseverance will be necessary.

Babies and toddlers show enormous amounts of perseverance in learning basic gross and fine motor skills like standing, walking, talking, learning to feed themselves, etc. As your child grows and develops though, so do the challenges they face. Beginning around three years old, your child's obstacles and challenges will move away from survival-based skills and will begin to expand to school, social and relationship, and sports and physical development challenges.

School

School can be a tough place to navigate for children. They evolve from one or two caregivers who are dedicated to their every whim and will into an environment in which they cannot demand to be taken care of. They delve into a world of different personalities, sharing, and learning, and certain expectations are placed on them to put in effort and produce results.

For younger kids, school is tough because it means having to deal with emotions, and as we know, young kids have giant feelings. Suddenly, your tiny tyke is charged with having to confront their own emotions and the emotions of others, and they will need to be taught how to persevere through their feelings to learn how to communicate their needs effectively.

Older children will be expected to complete homework that encompasses subjects outside of their particular interests, some of which they may not like.

Older children will need to learn that not persevering will ultimately lead to consequences, especially when it comes to their education and their grades. Kids who are taught to push through the homework and tasks they don't feel they're particularly great at, or don't like, will reap the rewards of better grade averages.

Social and Relationship

Because children are driven by impulsive, emotional decision-making, they can say things they don't mean. As your child grows they will become self-aware and will begin to develop a conscience. They will begin to realize that their words, as well as their actions, have the ability to hurt people and perseverance will help your kid to stand up and do the right thing by apologizing and learning from their mistakes.

This ability to humble oneself and admit to mistakes deepens relationships and solidifies their social standings in a group environment. Children should be taught to set aside their pride in moments where their actions have been hurtful and shown that avoiding the situation will not solve it.

Being shown that persevering through uncomfortable and difficult emotions and having the strength to do the right thing is hard—not just on emotional states of being, but mental states too. But, perseverance is incredibly important to forming and maintaining healthy relationships. It prevents bullying, and it helps children work through their own emotional and relationship issues, as well as developing empathy for the feelings of others.

Sports and Physical Activities

Aside from education, sports and physical activities require huge amounts of perseverance. Every person must have a tenacious, can-do attitude when they take on sports and physical activities in order for them to learn, develop, and hone their skills.

Kids have a fantastic fallback when they feel anything is too hard, and that fallback is avoidance. Children will tell you they are simply too busy or not interested in something purely because they lack the confidence or the perseverance to push their mind and body past discomfort.

Physical activity demands that a child understands Rome wasn't built in a day, and that sometimes they will need to push through a sore body and a tired mind to achieve something they have never done before.

What makes student athletes shine is a combination of passion and perseverance. Think about it, no amount of natural talent is going to make you push yourself harder to break your own records and achieve greatness.

Overcoming sore muscles, tiredness and fatigue requires your child to have the perseverance to push through their discomfort, and to remain focused on the goal at hand. It is the trait that drives kids to learn from their mistakes, brushing them off as nothing more than a learning curb, helping them to rise up to a challenge.

Most importantly, perseverance ensures kids are working with an intention not only to pursue their passion but to achieve whatever their definition of success is.

Remember, passion is the "why" behind your actions, whereas perseverance is the "how" to get it done.

How to Instill Perseverance in Kids

For parents to instill perseverance in their children, they need to have perseverance themselves.

Kids seem to fall into two distinct categories; the adventurous type and the cautious type. Children who are adventurous are somewhat easier to develop perseverance in because their naturally tenacious attitude will have them pushing their boundaries.

Cautious children or those with a lower self-esteem will need to have perseverance nurtured in them, and this will require you to be tenacious and patient in your approach.

As a parent, it is your responsibility to foster the traits of success in your child and your actions. How you choose to nurture your child will influence their ability to go into the world with passion and perseverance.

Let's look at some ways that you can help your child develop perseverance, especially if they are one of those kids who err on the side of caution.

Take notice of your child and what they are doing, and when you see your child persisting through something new or difficult, praise their effort. The point is to help your child see that their efforts are what gets the task done, not the outcome of their efforts. If your child is battling to tie their shoelaces and the end outcome is not quite what a tied shoe should look like, that's fine. Your child still deserves praise.

Always highlight why perseverance is important to them and to the people around them. Children don't have a natural sense of the advantages of perseverance. Kids need to know why they have to do things, it gives them a sense of purpose, and a reason to want to push through their discomfort.

Show up for your child, no matter what. You need to model perseverance and that means sticking to the things you have committed to. If you're half-hearted in your attempts to get things done, I guarantee you that your child will be too.

At every opportunity you can, show your child perseverance. This could be through news stories, people they admire, or even other kids. Sometimes children need to be shown the reward of perseverance rather than being told. Visual references are a great tool for kids, especially when they can reference this perseverance to people who are the same as them.

Your child may have a sense of how to set their own goals, but inexperienced goal-setters can sometimes do more harm than good because they have no idea how to break their goals down into smaller milestones. When goals are not broken down into smaller increments, they can appear to be unachievable, that's why helping your kid break their goals down will set themselves up for success.

Whenever you can, reframe things that they see as hard or difficult into something that is a valuable challenge. Kids need to know that nothing good comes out of avoidance, or half-heartedly completing tasks and that by persevering, they will have something to be proud of, regardless of the outcome of their efforts.

Fostering Perseverance in Cautious Kids

Cautious kids aren't just afraid of an outcome, they're actually afraid to try, and as parents, we hope that by telling our child to keep trying or to not give up, that our child will follow our instructions. Cautious kids, however, lack self-initiative because fear rules their decision-making processes. They would rather quit, or never try at all than have to deal with this fear.

But, fear can be broken down into many factors, and for you to foster perseverance in your cautious child, you will first need to understand what is driving their behavior.

Pressure—Both Internal and External

Kids are intuitive, they have to be to survive, and you will need to understand that the external pressure that you place on your child is internalized. When your child fails to meet your expectations, you are inadvertently telling them that they are not capable. This is especially true when effort is not praised.

Added to this, kids will often hurt themselves, or push the boundaries too far when they believe that they will only get your approval by submitting to the pressure placed on them. Let's look at an example:

Sam's son isn't just walking at 13 months, he is running. Your son has barely graduated to standing unsupported, let alone taking his first steps. You begin to encourage your son by holding their hand and dragging them along to push them to take their first steps. This leads to tumbles and falls that both scare and accidentally hurt your son. As a result, your child fears walking and takes longer to build enough confidence to take his first steps.

I know the above example is extreme, but sometimes our most well-intentioned actions can lead to external pressure that your child will inevitably internalize. When your kid fears that they will disappoint you by failing, they are less likely to even try a task at hand.

Children are not meant to be compared, they're meant to be nurtured as they grow at their own pace. If you are challenging your child with healthy stimuli, exposing them to new things, and praising their efforts, they will become resilient in their own way. Giving your child examples of perseverance should be about comparison, or rather about the act and reward of persevering.

When your cautious child tells you they can't do something it is usually a red flag that something deeper is going on. Listen to them, take a step back, and realize that you may be focusing on what you would like your child to achieve rather than the effort they are putting in.

Encourage effort, cheerleading your kid's bravery in trying. Avoid statements like, "I know you can do it," which are inadvertently pressurizing your child, because what happens if they really just aren't at a point where they can do it? Instead, use language that moves them away from pressure. "You tried so hard, that was amazing!"

Cautious children are different from those who are brave and curious. You can encourage being ready but ultimately they will only truly be ready when they have enough confidence to try and are no longer scared of failing you or those around them.

Helicopter Parenting

Parents can have a tendency to helicopter parent: being overly reactive, impulsively stopping their child from being curious, or over-responding to behaviors.

When parents choose this style of parenting they are subconsciously telling their child that they are not capable of doing things themselves. And I get it, no one wants to see their child get hurt, nor do they want their child to get into situations that are dangerous, but helicopter parenting is a primary source of an "I can't" attitude in children.

Here's the thing, if your child has climbed up onto the sofa, there is a pretty good chance that they know how to climb down, and even if they don't, they will figure it out. You constantly taking kids down is not going to teach them the skill of how to get down, nor is it going to allow them to develop the confidence required to learn how to get themselves out of the predicament they have put themselves in.

As parents, we need to wait and watch, and then wait and watch some more. You need to allow yourself and your child time to find out what they can do independently before stepping in to help them. And even when you step in, your child should first know that you are available to help, and not that you will swoop in to save them.

If you have already engaged in a lot of helicopter parenting behaviors, you're going to have some work to do to change your own attitude to help your child build their confidence. Instead of hopping in to help your child, let them know that it is better if they try to help themselves first. Let your child know that you are there to keep them safe and to offer them guidance but insist that they try, with minimal help, and then praise their efforts.

"Could you hold onto the side of the wall and put one foot down on the step below? Well done! Let's try another step."

Having Negative Associations and Experiences

When children have had negative experiences or experienced trauma surrounding certain activities, their fear may be paralyzing.

Trauma is incredibly powerful and your child will need to know that letting go as much as they possibly can, within safe confines, will help them to develop courage and perseverance. Don't try to go in for the hard sell when your child has experienced trauma or has had a negative experience.

Rather, let them know that you acknowledge their feelings and their fears, and help them to understand that together, you can help them to overcome whatever is holding them back.

It is important to not push your child outside of their comfort zone when there has been trauma. Make it incredibly clear that the power is in their hands to stop whenever they feel like everything feels too much.

Trauma demands that you take baby steps with your child without helicopter parenting them so that they can see that they are capable of overcoming their trauma.

External Stressors

External stressors can change a usually confident, adventurous child into a cautious one. When a child who is normally confident starts to think "I can't do it" they have probably experienced something fairly recently that has made them feel unsafe or unconfident in their own abilities.

Changes like moving cities or homes, a new sibling, or moving schools can trigger a sudden lack of perseverance in your child.

Parents need to take a step back and assess what is happening in their kid's life. Find out what your child needs help with and understand that transition requires help as well. It's not enough to reframe external stressors as your child will know that this is only being said to placate them.

Instead, you need to acknowledge how they are feeling and that they are going through a tough time. Ask them how you can help them get through whatever it is they are experiencing. Don't try to coax your kid into changing back to their normal persevering self.

Most of all, don't judge them for their current behavior and praise their efforts when they dip their toes back into adventure and curiosity.

Combating Frustration

Frustration requires a different kind of perseverance because frustration is driven by anger, not fear.

When a child battles to overcome a task, or when they have to battle their own wants and needs because they can't have something, it can take perseverance to come out the other side and do what is right.

Kids have a considerable amount of milestones they need to achieve outside of basic functions like walking and talking. Riding a bicycle, tying their shoelaces, and learning to brush their teeth are all just a tiny fraction of things your child needs to master throughout their childhood.

Adults get frustrated too; we get angry, may feel despair, or even discouraged when things don't work out in the way we expect them to, but for kids, frustration can be an overwhelming situation.

Introducing your children to new skills and obstacles that will inevitably lead to frustration is a good way to teach them how to overcome frustration. When you help your child see that frustration is an inevitable part of life, and that learning to overcome it is a valuable skill to have in life, you set your child up for success.

You will need to assess what your child's general temperament is in order to best help them overcome their frustrations. Some kids will become frustrated and dissolve into tears, others will lash out by screaming and shouting, while others may even begin to laugh or become quiet.

Once you know what your child's go-to reaction is to frustration, you can ascertain what level of frustration your child is experiencing. Levels of frustration can vary depending on how difficult the task at hand is, what expectations your child has, and what your child wants to achieve through completing the task.

Frustration that is not dealt with and addressed correctly can be extremely damaging to your child's self-esteem. Think about this, "I'm not good at this." is only a step away from, "I'm not good." or "I'm not good at anything."

Every time your child undertakes new tasks, they will learn to incorporate three steps in order for them to be successful in their endeavors.

They will need to learn how to self-soothe and master their frustration. This will teach them patience and will help them to develop self-control and self-calming behaviors. You can certainly suggest some strategies for your child to overcome their frustrations, but ultimately what you need to do is help your kid to identify that they are frustrated and that they can control how they act and react to their frustration.

They will overcome their frustration and begin to believe in their capabilities. When your child pushes through their frustration, they build their self-worth and start to believe in the process of learning a new skill. They begin to rely less on their strengths and more on their determination and what they have learned by trying. This helps them to unravel what they need to tweak and change to improve the next time they try the same task.

They begin to see the value in trial and error. Your child now knows that they will experience frustration when trying something new, and will either choose to put themselves through the frustration again, or they will choose to avoid tasks that create frustration because either the reward was not self-gratifying enough, or that they don't believe there is any value in trying again.

Instead of diverting your child's attention when they are frustrated, wait and observe before you act to help your child. Let your child know that forever is a long time to not try amazing new things.

Empower your kid by allowing them to consider solutions to their frustration, and understand that small milestones for you are huge milestones for your child. Let them know that you see and acknowledge their frustration, and help them see that frustration is only a short step away from determination.

Chapter 5:

Strategy 4—

Conscientiousness

"What we accomplish in the marathon of life depends tremendously on our grit—our passion and perseverance for long-term goals." — Angela Duckworth

Did you know that children who are conscientious, and who have an adventurous, curious spirit are four times more likely to be academically successful (Bergold., et al. 2018)?

In the past, it was thought that conscientiousness and a sense of adventure were linked to personality traits, but these qualities can be nurtured and grown in children.

Parents of children who are naturally methodical, and who push themselves through each task with grit find it a little easier to nurture this trait in their kids. But, for parents who have children that are less conscientious, their child's casual, relaxed attitude about life can be frustrating.

Why Kids Need Conscientiousness

Being conscientious requires a person to perform tasks or to approach life with a thorough, vigilant approach. People who are conscientious take on each task they are given with patience and to the best of their ability. They seem to understand that rushing or taking shortcuts only leads to more work being done because the outcome will not be the desired one.

People who work conscientiously tend to be more organized and only have to complete a task once, making them far more efficient than their sometimes chaotic counterparts.

When combined with curiosity, kids are able to approach new tasks with an open mind and can work through these new tasks with diligence and a can-do attitude. They embrace anything new because they know that by approaching it with a methodical, conscientious approach, they will complete the task to the best of their ability.

Natural Conscientiousness Versus Taught Conscientiousness

As I have mentioned, it was thought that conscientiousness was more about personality than it was a taught skill. Newer research however, shows that personality is 50% inherent, and 50% learned.

What this means for your child is that while they may be somewhat chaotic at times, they can still be taught to be conscientious in their approach to life.

Good news, isn't it?

Even better news is that the smallest changes in a person's learned personality traits can create huge positive ripples in a person's career, happiness, relationships, and life in general.

All of this means that personalities can change as people grow and get older. When a child is taught to be organized and disciplined in their approach to life, and when these lessons are consistently taught, conscientiousness can become part of even the most chaotic personalities.

Many of the changes that need to be made for you to instill conscientiousness in your child will begin with placing a lot of emphasis on the benefits of being organized as well as how not being conscientious affects your child. There are some other small steps you can begin with right now to help your child become more conscientious.

Help your child recognize when they are acting chaotically and don't shy away from assisting your child in recognizing negative behaviors. Focus should always be placed on your child's behaviors and not on their personality.

Start small when asking your child to become more conscientious. You cannot expect your usually chaotic child to become organized overnight. Let them choose what they would like to become more organized in, and then help them find out what forms of organization works best for them. Once they have the hang of one organizational skill, move on to the next.

Practice patience with your child and recognize when they are intentionally trying to be conscientious in their tasks. Remember that grit and a growth mindset requires focus to be placed on effort, not success. If your child has managed to keep their bedroom neat, tidy, and organized for a week rather than three days, that is the progress made.

Fostering Conscientiousness

Older children can be easier to teach conscientiousness because they know and experience the consequences of not being conscientious. Older kids understand the value of working with diligence and determination.

Most younger kids naturally show lower levels of conscientiousness even if their levels of curiosity and adventure are a lot higher than older children. Younger children can be taught conscientiousness pretty easily though, and it doesn't take much effort because younger children want to be helpful.

For younger kids, teaching conscientiousness can be done by:

Giving your children age-appropriate chores and praising their efforts in completing their chores.

Allowing them to help you out with "grown-up tasks" like washing fruit and vegetables, helping to carry in groceries, etc.

Setting clear, concise boundaries.

Modeling conscientious behavior.

Giving feedback on their conscientious behavior and brainstorming how they believe they can or should improve.

Clearly define right and wrong in terms of your family morals and values.

Point out acts of conscientiousness, especially during storytimes.

Young children shouldn't be bribed and rewarded with physical rewards like toys, candy, or even an allowance. The aim is to teach your child that conscientiousness has its own reward, which is pride. Allowances and other rewards should be reserved for additional tasks completed to instill a sense of work ethic in your child.

Conscientiousness encourages your child to act responsibly and when combined with perseverance, kids learn to take these responsibilities seriously. Kids who are taught to be conscientious are more likely to try, try, and try again which is an invaluable skill to have when you consider how much they still have to learn in their life.

It is critical when teaching your child to be conscientious to help your child see that the process of completing a task is just as important as the completion. Do encourage curiosity and a sense of adventure but make sure that your child doesn't develop a wishy-washy attitude to life—conscientiousness is about commitment to the process and seeing a task through to its completion.

Instill problem-solving and decision-making abilities in your child so that they are invested in the choices they make to be conscientious.

Time Management and Communication in Conscientiousness

Like adults, kids may feel that they just don't have the time to be diligent and conscientious in completing their tasks. Children must learn, just like their adult counterparts, that much of conscientiousness has to do with remaining motivated to complete the task at hand. This is why kids need to be rewarded in ways that encourage internal motivation rather than money and gifts.

But no amount of self-motivation is going to keep your child motivated to complete a task properly if they have convinced themselves they don't have the time, or if they simply don't know how to manage their time effectively. And let's face it, time management is not a strength most children possess, nor do they know how to express that they can't manage their time.

It is a parent's responsibility to help your child assign the right amount of time to the tasks they have been assigned and break these tasks down into specific time measurable milestones.

Observe how your child uses their time when assigned tasks and then set them up for success by showing them where they can save time, and then help them set up a schedule or daily planner. Include them when you evaluate their daily planner, showing them where they used their time effectively. Show your child the value of completing their responsibilities and tasks conscientiously, highlighting how much time they have gained for fun stuff by completing a task properly the first time.

Finally, model proper communication with your child. Let your kid talk to you about how they feel about their allotted times, and whether they believe it is enough time for the task at hand. As kids grow they will need more time for some tasks and less for others. When a child can communicate their time needs it is easier for all parties involved to come to compromises that work for everyone.

Younger children should be encouraged to be helpful rather than labeling them as not conscientious. Kids under ten years old have a very limited perspective of what being helpful is, and when you show them what they can do to help you, conscientiousness is developed naturally.

Focus on self-motivation and praise positive responses from your children. Kids need to help out from a place of desire to be useful rather than being instructed to help. In other words, your children should not feel like pawns in the chess game of your life's responsibilities and duties. Rather, they should feel like an integral part of a family unit where their contribution is helpful and needed.

Accept your child's type of help and don't correct them.

Let them help you with the little things so that they feel important too.

Prepare for the possibility that tasks completed to your child's best ability may not align with your expectations. It's about effort, not expectation, and practice makes perfect. Your child will get better at the tasks assigned to them as time goes on.

Conscientiousness and Creativity

A lot of focus is placed on academics to foster qualities of diligence and conscientiousness, but creativity and openness are incredibly useful tools to use in creating a conscientious child.

Change is scary, even for adults, and the bottom line is that even the most creative minds will tell you that change is more of an evolutionary process, especially when creativity is lacking.

True visionaries however, who work diligently towards achieving their goals are extremely creative. Creativity may not seem like it is a particularly conscientious practice though, especially when creative people are often labeled as messy and chaotic.

But, when we break down the creative process, it becomes apparent that creativity and uniqueness go hand in hand with conscientiousness.

Preparation—The stage in which information is gathered and a person researches, dreams, and conceives what it is they would like to achieve by trying something new.

Incubation—When the mind makes a decision to participate in something new and begins to imagine the possible outcomes.

Illumination—The moment in which the brain has its eureka moment and all of the imagined outcomes, as well as the paths to these outcomes, come to an actionable solution. This stage may seem messy to outsiders but in actuality, it is an act of conscientiousness, sifting through ideas and finding a solution.

Implementation—All of the previous stages are placed into action, and the creativity or new task begins to take shape.

When we unpack creativity and newness this way, it is pretty clear how conscientiousness is required for children to be creative. But creativity doesn't get enough of the spotlight when it comes to fostering conscientiousness in children, but it will be one of your greatest allies by allowing them to tame their chaos and become conscientious by tapping into their creativity.

Let's look at some ways in which you can develop and nurture your child's creative, open, mind so that you can help your child turn to conscientiousness naturally.

Encourage What-If Scenarios

Kids who are encouraged to ask what-if questions are more likely to turn to a problem-solving mentality when dealing with new tasks and activities that require conscientiousness. Children who ask or are asked what-if questions are more likely to be able to develop methods in which they can find solutions to issues they are facing and will be able to implement milestones to help solve problems and tackle tasks.

Find Creative Solutions to Mistakes

Mistakes happen, and being conscientious requires people to examine these mistakes— finding creative, new solutions to correct the issues at hand. But we often dismiss our children's creative solutions as nothing more than excuses. The reality is that your child's creative mind is working through the solutions at hand and it's up to you to decode their thoughts and help them to implement their ideas.

Build Upon Your Child's Interests

Conscientiousness needs to build slowly with small steps to make big changes in your child's life. This is far easier when you build upon your child's current interests by introducing new challenges along the way. If your child is great at painting, introduce them to pastels and allow them to figure out how they can be creative with a new medium. Or, if your child is great at dancing, introduce them to martial arts in which they can move their body differently. This teaches children how to become conscientious in all tasks so that they can improve in their life, rather than only sticking with the things they feel that they are naturally talented in.

Avoid Asking Your Child Closed-Ended Questions

Open-ended questions provoke discussion and creative thought. When you ask your child open-ended questions, it's as if they are asking themselves the questions. Open-ended questions help form ideas whereas closed-ended questions have a finite yes or no answer.

Open-ended questions encourage your child to conscientiously prepare for not only the desired outcome, but all other imagined situations.

Let's look at an example of this:

"You have told me you are going for a hike on Saturday. What might happen if the weather changes unexpectedly during the hike?"

Asking your child a question in this way helps them to think of all eventualities, and ensures that they pack and prepare properly for their hike.

If you asked your child the question in a different way like, "Have you prepared for weather changes?" they are less likely to think of how they could prepare and will probably answer with a simple yes or no.

Spend Time With Your Child Throughout Their Creative Process

Parents have a tendency to want to know an outcome rather than sitting through their child's creative process. Spend time with your child as they sift through each of their possible solutions, and hear them out as they make their decisions.

By being with your child throughout their creative process you are able to develop a plan with them that factors in time management, as well as conscientious milestones that help them to work toward their goals.

Schedule Creative Time

Creativity is as important as academics and athletic achievements. Creativity improves cognitive function and problem-solving skills, and for kids who lack creativity, conscientiousness can be difficult.

Kids should have time set aside for unstructured creative time in which they can explore their inner creativity and conscientiously create outside of structured academic programs and organized activities.

Always remember that creativity can be broadly defined and it is important to allow your child to be creative based on their own ideas.

Encourage Risk-Taking When it Comes to Creativity

When your kid comes home with a creative project, it is important to encourage them to think outside of the box, even if they aren't sure of what the outcome will be when they complete the task.

Allow your child to express their vision, and ask them what steps they will take to reach their desired outcome. Once your child has decided what they will do to achieve their desired result, follow their creative process. Let them work diligently through the steps they have outlined for themselves but don't stifle their creativity if they need to go back to the drawing board to think of other creative ideas in order for them to conscientiously complete their task.

Creativity not only improves your child's cognitive functions but is also the foundation of conscientiousness. Science shows that people who take time to be creative as a habit have stronger links between the hemispheres of their brain (Shi et al., 2017).

It helps to develop new neural connections and facilitates new ideas which in turn allows kids to learn perseverance as part of their personality.

Aside from that, creativity helps to stabilize people's moods, and therapists have long turned to creative movement and activities to help self-regulation and develop attention spans.

Continued Conscientiousness

Studies show that conscientiousness dips when kids become teenagers. This is especially true for teenage boys, who have quite a significant change in their ability to be conscientious (Jarrett, 2018). A mixture of hormones and the changes that occur in a teenager's frontal cortex all play a part in this change, and for parents who had previously very conscientious kids, this sudden flip in behavior can be quite disconcerting.

Teenagers need to be treated with kid gloves when it comes to conscientiousness, and while some of the tools I have already laid out for you may work, others will just have your teen pushing back and descending further into chaos.

The most important aspect of conscientiousness you can help your teen with is time management, allowing them enough time for themselves as a reward for working conscientiously. Aside from this though, there are other tools, tips, and tricks that you can use to help reignite conscientiousness in your teenagers.

Let Your Teen Know They Have the Power to Make Good Decisions

Teenagers tend to lean toward risky behavior, usually as a way to feel socially included. As parents, we spend so much time trying to tell our teens what they should or shouldn't do that we neglect to let our teens know that they are equipped with everything they need to make good decisions. And just because your teen is becoming more independent, doesn't mean that they don't need to know that you are still a safe space to bounce ideas off of, or the person they can turn to when they are in a tough situation.

Model Empathy and Kindness

It's easy to become frustrated and angry with teenagers, especially when their behaviors become questionable or when your once loving, sweet child, has turned into a surly half-adult.

Modeling empathy and kindness, especially when your teen is going through a tough time, will help them think about their actions. People are less likely to lash out and be nasty to those who are kind to them, and when you have a teen who is calm and rational, you are more likely to be able to have a meaningful conversation with them about their choices and behaviors.

Trust Your Teen To Be Safe, But Be Aware

You certainly don't need to monitor everything your teenager does, but you do need to be aware of what is going on in their life, and you do need to put reasonable precautions in place. Conscientiousness requires a level of self-discipline, and with your teen being tempted by so many external influences, it is your job to keep them safe from themselves.

Removing temptations, or at the very least, discussing these temptations and the consequences of them should be done often. Try not to lecture your teen though, and make sure that you highlight the benefits of working conscientiously through the things they have to do so that they have the time to do the things they want to do.

Keep Them Safe From the Blue Light Trap

One of the biggest thieves of modern times is technology. Social media, gaming, texting, and streaming services will become a large part of your teen's life. You will need to teach your child how to be responsible online, not just from a safety point of view, but from a time-management point of view.

Teenagers, especially, need to understand and learn to appreciate how conscientiousness can benefit their life. But teenagers cannot be told what to do, and sometimes it can feel like you're running repeatedly into a brick wall when trying to show your teen the right way to do things.

For you to get through to your teen, and for your teen to understand why conscientiousness is important you will need to really highlight the benefits of doing things properly the first time around.

If Nothing Else, Be Conscientious

Kids who are conscientious are often seen as dependable to their peers because they have the ability to self-regulate and control their behaviors, and teachers who are conscientious often produce kids who have higher levels of productivity and higher average grades.

Why?

Conscientiousness is the cautious approach to working diligently through tasks. It takes into account not only the behaviors required to complete a task but also the effects of the outcome of this task on others and yourself. Conscientiousness consists of six traits that drive certain behaviors. These six traits include process-orientation, caution, organization, self-discipline, a sense of duty, and self-motivation.

When we look at these traits, it begins to make sense that conscientious people are more likely to succeed as they focus on the processes at hand so that each sub-task can be completed properly. As a child begins to see that conscientious work yields successful results, they tend to push to achieve higher goals.

But conscientiousness is not diving into a task head first to complete each of the steps required for success. When we look at conscientious people there is an element of caution. Often this caution is seen as consideration, or planning ahead, and while this step may seem irrelevant it is actually a big part of being conscientious.

Let's say your child has an essay due in five days, you're frustrated because they have not begun the essay yet and a day has passed. After discussing this with your child you realize they have a process and that what you thought was laziness and procrastination is all part of being a conscientious worker. Your child has plotted out the information they require, sourced the information, and broken down each section of the essay into how much needs to be written every day for the next four days.

Once your conscientious child puts the plan into action and achieves each of their milestones, successfully achieving a completed essay is inevitable.

If nothing else, your child should be encouraged to be conscientious in what they do because being conscientious will ultimately mean they try new things, set higher goals, and will be self-motivated to complete their tasks according to the steps they have set out for themselves.

While conscientiousness is required to be gritty, grit is a byproduct of being conscientious. If kids are taught to work conscientiously, they will ignite their passions, and will work with a purpose toward achieving their goals. Children who are conscientious are more likely to be resilient because they have thought through their processes and have considered the pros and cons, and as we all know, resilience is wholeheartedly needed for your child to succeed in a tough world.

Chapter 6:

Strategy 5—Resilience

"Nobody wants to show you the hours and hours of becoming. They'd rather show the highlight of what they've become."— Angela Duckworth

Kids have a built-in ability to work through the many challenges they face and can cope with the normal, age-appropriate stresses and strains of life. Parents, however, try to shield their children from these normal obstacles and, as a result, remove our children's confidence to overcome problems as well as their ability to bounce back from failures and adversity.

Children will need to learn to be resilient if they are to cope in a tough adult world, and teaching your child to be courageous, curious, and passionate about the world around them will all be for nothing if your child doesn't have the resilience to come back from failure.

You see, children should be allowed to be brave, curious, and even trusting of their natural instincts.Resilience ensures that they can step outside of their comfort zone when they are ready to push the limits of what they have already learned.

Why Kids Need to Be Resilient

If you are going to have a child who works conscientiously toward their goals, they will need to develop resilience.

Resilience ensures that your child looks at each mistake they have made and problems they encounter as something to overcome. It allows your child to make the decision independently, and to stand up, dust themselves off, and take a step forward when they are faced with failure.

Because children will face stress in some way. shape, or form as they grow, resilience gives your child the wherewithal to "toughen up" and deal with their issues, or if the issue is too large to deal with themselves, to put their pride aside to seek guidance from an adult.

While some of the obstacles kids face might seem insignificant to adults, for kids, they can be overwhelming if they don't possess the resilience to analyze what went wrong and how they can move forward.

Where courage helps your child to look fear in the eye, resilience will have your kid confronting their problems, stepping forward rather than remaining stagnant or retreating to safety.

And, the more your child learns to deal with their problems, the easier it becomes for them to bounce back and confront other issues in their life in a way that is healthy. Resilience is your child's inner voice that tells them that they are strong enough and capable enough to handle kid-sized problems and that they are smart enough to know when the problem is too big for them to handle on their own.

How to Build Resilience in Your Child

As a parent, you can help your child become resilient and show them how confronting their problems is a good way to solve issues independently.

When you, as an adult, jump in to help your child avoid problems, or when you solve their problems for them, you are weakening their resilience, and as a result, you are weakening their ability to cope with the challenges life throws at them.

Without resilience, kids find it difficult to tap into their natural, creative problem-solving capabilities, and ultimately, kids who are not allowed to be resilient, will end up anxious, avoidant, and shut down from the rest of the world.

Many of the strategies listed for courage, conscientiousness, and perseverance will automatically develop resilience, but sometimes kids need a little bit of an extra push to become independent and resilient.

Emotionally Connect With Your Child

So much of your child's resilience depends on a strong emotional connection with the adults in their life. Kids need to learn to be confident, but even the most confident of people sometimes need a soft place to fall.

Children want to test their boundaries in a way that is safe for them and by spending one-on-one time with your child and developing a deeper emotional connection, you are saying to your kid that they are free to explore the world around them while knowing they will be safe from any real danger.

This means that you will have to put down that phone, cancel your engagements, and actually spend time with your kid and watch how they interact with the world around them. Your child needs to know that they have your love and support as they adventure and explore and that you will keep them safe should they step too far outside of their comfort zone.

And, as your child grows older, they will know that they have someone who is mature and engaged enough in their life to seek out support and guidance in times when they feel the situation they are facing requires a more experienced viewpoint.

Good positive connections with your child will show them the value of relationships and unification when times are tough, and the best kind of resilience is knowing that sometimes teamwork makes the dream work.

Your Child Needs to Know You Will Keep Them Safe When it Counts

There was a time when kids were allowed to be kids, and playgrounds weren't lined with soft flooring and foam edges. While these things are all put in place to ensure no real harm is done to a child, it has kind of become a metaphor for modern parenting.

You cannot keep your child safe all of the time, and even if you could, this would result in mentally and physically weak individuals who would have a really tough time trying to survive adulthood. And no parent wants their child to purely survive once they are grown—the point of life is to thrive!

Children have to be taught to take healthy risks in life for them to be able to explore life outside of their comfort zone. Preventing your child from trying that new, but slightly risky sport, or speaking to someone new, is not a real risk to their life. Parents who enable their children to avoid taking risks are only stunting their growth and destroying their kid's self-esteem.

Kids need to know that they can embrace taking risks and that if they push too far, that you will intervene.

Stop Fixing Your Child's Problems

It is normal for children to come to their parents to help them to fix the issues in their life, and it is even more normal for parents to go straight into a corrective mode, lecturing and explaining how issues should be resolved.

The issue with your child solving issues this way is that they're actually not solving the issue at all—they're expecting you to do the hard part. When kids aren't allowed the opportunity to solve their own issues, they feel lost and confused and ultimately, they will spend their lives relying on others to overcome even the smallest of challenges for them.

But, we don't want to turn our kids away when they come to us for guidance, so how do you deal with the situation when your child comes to you for help?

Tap into your child's creative mind!

Ask your child questions and allow them to bounce solutions off of you so that they can understand that they're capable of solving some problems themselves. Helping your child think their way through to the other side of the issues they are facing helps them to build resilience, not reliance, and ultimately a sense of responsibility for issues they can solve alone.

Problem-Solving Skills Are Really Important

Nothing builds and promotes resilience like the ability to turn inward to analyze and problem-solve pertinent issues. And yes, we all need help from time to time, but it is important for kids to know that they can be self-reliant too.

Teach your kids how to brainstorm solutions, and how to present these solutions in a way that will be beneficial to all parties. When parents are open to listening to a child's problem-solving process they are encouraging kids to first turn inward and then outward when dealing with problems.

Added to this, a problem-solving, brainstorming mindset means your child will always find a responsible adult to discuss bigger problems with, ensuring that you never need to interrogate your child to find out what issues they are facing and how they are dealing with them.

Label Issues, Not Behaviors

Naming emotions may be tough for kids, but labeling issues can be even tougher. This is because kids can sometimes feel overwhelmed by even the smallest of issues, and teaching them to label and categorize their issues will help them know which metaphorical box to refer to in their minds to find the solutions.

Ask your child about the issue they are facing and how they are feeling so that you can assist label the issue, and then let them problem-solve their way through it. It's important to let your child choose the labels of their 'boxes' so that they know how to reference their issues in the future.

Make sure to have an "adult issue" label as well so that your child doesn't try to deal with issues they shouldn't be dealing with on their own like inappropriate touch, severe bullying, moral dilemma, life-endangering situations, etc.

Kids build resilience through self-confidence, and self-confidence comes easier to those children who believe they are capable of not just solving their problems, but that they will come through the other side stronger than they were before.

Teach Them Coping Skills

Kids need to know how to self-soothe and pull themselves out of their mood so that they can be in the right state of mind to solve their problems.

Help your child identify the difference between emotions, feelings, and mood, and let them know that they have the power to change how they feel and the mood they are in. When kids feel empowered and understand that they don't have to be a victim of their feelings, they are more likely to want to approach issues with a level head. And, when your child starts to take on issues with a level-headed approach, they are increasing their chances of successfully solving their own issues.

Resilience demands a level head, and the ability to not wallow in negative feelings and moods. The goal is to get through life's issues with a positive can-do attitude, not a "why does life keep happening to me" stance.

Promote Positivity

Hindsight is a wonderful thing because it allows us to find the blessings and lessons we learned from the hardships in our lives.

What if I told you that you would never need hindsight if you tackled life's challenges with a positive mindset when you were facing the storm?

Promoting positivity in your child helps them become the eye of the storm, providing calmness and respite while they are dealing with problems. A positive mindset ensures that your kid understands that every mistake and every situation comes with a choice to throw their hands up in defeat or to anchor themselves to drive through to the other side.

We are all going to face issues in life, and sometimes life will happen to us, so teach your child to have an attitude that allows them to appreciate what life has given them rather than be a hopeless passenger.

When people have a positive mindset, resilience comes naturally because they know with absolute certainty that they shape the outcome, regardless of what is happening around them.

Take Your Kid Outside

After being restricted to indoor life for the better part of two years as the world endured a global pandemic, the value of being outdoors has once again been placed in the spotlight.

From mental health benefits to the physical benefits of being in the fresh air, children, and in fact, all people, need to be outside. Being outside will activate your child's imagination, curiosity, and sense of adventure. It will trigger their biological instincts to push their limits, and when they do, you will need to take a step back and let them.

That's right, if your child is not in immediate danger of severely injuring themselves or others, you will need to stand aside, observe, and only guide them when it is asked of you. Let your child struggle so that they can see what they are capable of, and then encourage them to try, try, and try again.

The 7 Cs of Resilience

Pediatrician and human development expert, Dr. Kenneth Ginsburg has theorized that there are seven ingredients to reliance, especially in children.

These ingredients are: competence, connection, contribution, control, coping, confidence, and character.

To build resilience in children, each of these seven cs should be carefully worked on to ensure that your child becomes responsibly resilient.

1. Competence

Competence will help your child deal with stress effectively. When a child is competent, they have been equipped with the correct skills to overcome issues and challenges and know how to apply these skills. In other words, competence is the ability to competently deal with the situation at hand.

Kids need to be competent in a variety of situations in their life, and it's important that you help your child understand the difference between knowing how to overcome their issues and actually implementing the skills you have taught them.

Competence reduces stress, improves social interactions, and gives your kid the opportunity to effectively manage issues independently.

Give your child an opportunity to practice the skills you have taught them so that they can develop their competence in problem-solving.

2. Connection

Kids need to feel like they are closely connected to their friends and family. Children who have a close connection to their community have a much stronger sense of safety and belonging.

Developing your child's sense of connection will ensure that a great set of values are instilled in them, negating self-destructive and other negative behaviors.

Parents need to foster a deeper, more meaningful relationship with their kids, and to introduce them to other adults who are safe, nurturing, and inspiring.

This teaches your child empathy and helps them develop strong emotional ties of their own growing up, making them a good friend, a great member of a family, and develops them into useful community members.

3. Contribution

Everyone wants to feel like they belong and that they are contributing to the world around them.

Children who learn to contribute to the world positively understand that acts of service have a ripple effect, and that small actions have the potential to create great change.

Teach your child that they don't need to do huge things to make a difference—being polite, saying thank you, and smiling all have the ability to change someone else's day. Don't forget to do the same when your child contributes, as they will be more willing to contribute to the home and to your requests if they feel they are valued.

This willingness to help will improve their competence in completing tasks, as they practice these tasks over and over again, and will strengthen their sense of connection to you.

Explore the concept of contribution with your child by discussing how they believe they contribute to their own lives, their family life, and to the people they are in touch with daily.

4. Control

Children need to be taught that they have complete control over their actions, feelings, and decisions. Kids who are taught that they have control over their lives are more likely to make the right decisions and to accept the mistakes they have made.

Kids need to be exposed to choices and to be able to experience the consequences of these choices. Resilience requires repetition of actions to become good at what needs to be done but also the ability to overcome mistakes and problems. Kids who know how to control their actions are able to bounce back from mistakes quicker.

5. Coping

When kids are exposed to a wide range of coping skills in all categories, they learn how to cope with the stresses and strains of their life.

Children need to know how to reduce their stress levels, how to manage situations in the moment, and when to turn to an adult for assistance or guidance. Coping skills are critical in developing resilience as children will feel that they are better equipped to deal with situations that others may feel are overwhelming.

6. Confidence

Confident kids believe in their ability to face life and to thrive while doing so. Children gain confidence through numerous means but ultimately, having parents who enable good behavior, facing real-life challenges, and an ability to think outside the box when it comes to solution-finding, will grow a child's confidence.

When children are confident, they learn to become self-motivated, and understand that by putting their mind to the task at hand, and pushing through diligently will yield the best outcome for them.

Confident children are resilient children because they have a belief in themselves and their ability to do whatever they want to do.

7. Character

Children who are allowed to develop their own character have a stronger sense of self, including confidence and self-worth. When a child's behavior is focused on rather than their character, you are more likely to reinforce that you respect their values but not their current behavior.

Kids with a strong sense of their character tend to make wiser decisions and feel a deeper need to contribute positively in their own lives and in the lives of others. And, when a child has great self-esteem they become resilient because they don't allow challenges to keep them down.

Resilience is important in life. It helps kids overcome adversity and strife and equips them with the skills they need to tackle small and big issues. People cope with frustration and issues differently, but resilience is the ability to look at a situation, and identify the risks, the process, and the outcome.

Being resilient doesn't mean your child will never experience stressful or emotional situations in their life. Resilience is the ability to overcome this stress and to deal with the emotions they are feeling.

Teaching your child to be resilient will show them how to be adaptable and flexible when facing issues, and will help them understand that hard work and diligence trumps intelligence every single time.

Resilient children are happy children. They look at every challenge and tasks they're faced with as a moment to grow and learn. They manage their frustration and self-regulate how they feel so that they can set emotions aside for a problem-solving, rational thought process.

Chapter 7:

Summarizing How to Develop Grit and Resilience

"Most dazzling human achievements are, in fact, the aggregate of countless individual elements, each of which is, in a sense, ordinary."—Angela Duckworth

Studies have shown that academic, athletic, and balanced success in students have less to do with intelligence and more to do with the grit of the child. Kids who showed high levels of grittiness, who were ambitious, and practiced self-control, were far more likely to do better in school and displayed higher levels of intelligence (Duckworth, 2015).

Since Duckworth's original studies back in 2007, other research has been done which shows just how critical grit is in children. Almost all of these subsequent studies have shown that perseverance, grit, passion, resilience, and empathy are far more important than a child's IQ when it comes to academic performance.

But parents can be a huge stumbling block in a child's ability to become gritty and resilient. These studies show that parents expect more of their same sex children—mothers expect their daughters to be tougher, while fathers expect their sons to be grittier, and this means ultimately one parent will end up overly protective of their child.

This overprotective instinct is counterintuitive and in no way builds grit in kids. Children need to become frustrated and struggle to complete tasks in order for them to learn. Mistakes need to be made for them to find out how to do things properly, and while it might seem counterintuitive, it's only through mistakes that we learn what the next best step is.

Ultimately, challenges are a part of life, and taking risks is the only way people progress. Because kids are still learning all of the things they need to become functional adults, almost everything will be a struggle or a challenge.

What parents should be paying attention to is how anxious a child becomes as they navigate their way through a new challenge, offering them coping mechanisms rather than assisting them in completing the task. Kids who are helped in everything they do will only learn that someone else can and will do their hard tasks for them, and will ultimately fall behind their grittier peers.

Be prepared though! Kids will complain, become angry, cry, and even throw things around when they become frustrated during new tasks. Tasks that are age-appropriate need to be tried over and over again for your child to learn, and stepping in to help your child is ultimately more damaging than good. This doesn't mean you need to leave your kid to kick and scream through newness, as this in itself can be damaging, and will teach your child that newness is scary and frustrating.

Instead, offer the right kind of help by instilling problem-solving skills, having discussions with them, and helping them learn coping skills for frustration.

By always jumping to your child's aid, you are denying them a full life in which they experience frustration but also feel a sense of greatness and capability.

Recapping a Growth Mindset

People who have a growth mindset are naturally far more resilient. This is because they are more focused on the task at hand, rather than the outcome. I'm not saying that these people don't work with an end goal in mind, but they understand that working hard and with purpose in the present will facilitate the end goal as a byproduct.

When kids are raised to have a growth mindset, they push through challenges because they know that to struggle at times is part and parcel of overall success. They have a deeper belief that failure is never a permanent state, nor do they believe that they will not come through the issues they are facing.

Remember that a growth mindset is necessary for your child to build grit because they need to understand that anything is possible with determination and the right amount of work. Kids need to acknowledge that they have both strengths and weaknesses, but that weaknesses are not an indication that they cannot do something. It just means you have to try harder from time to time.

For kids to have a growth mindset, adults need to focus less on talent and more on a child's ability to go through the processes of learning something new. In addition, the adults in a child's life need to actually model the behavior they want to see, and that means taking on tasks that are challenging for them too.

Adopting a growth mindset may be a challenge itself for parents though, as most were raised to believe that working within their strengths was the only way to succeed. Because of this, parents need to be thoughtful, deliberate, and inspiring in the words they choose when coaching their child toward a growth mindset.

You want to be able to talk to your kids about the true meaning of greatness and about the processes of working within their purpose, passions, and beliefs. It's important that your child understands that the world demands uniqueness and a variety of skills as well as creative thinkers and doers.

Growth mindsets are developed on behaviors rather than talents, and it is vitally important that you shy away from highlighting how intelligent or naturally talented your child is. Instead of saying, "You're so smart, just look at these grades," you should say, "I can see that you really applied yourself and studied hard to achieve these grades." Because when it comes down to it, natural talent can only take a person so far in their life before they plateau, and if you never teach your child how to work hard, they will never achieve their personal greatness.

Children need to understand that success is always in the effort they put in rather than the talents they are blessed with.

The Changes You Need to Make For Your Child

As parents and childminders, we will need to make some changes in our behaviors so that we can model the right behaviors for our children. Because kids learn more from what they see than what they hear, it is important that you are not just saying the right things but are actually doing the right things.

1. Show Your Child That Difficult Things Can Be Learned

Take on tasks that you feel are challenging and discuss with your child how you are dealing with these challenges. When teaching your child that difficult tasks can be learned it is important not to just model what you are saying but to actually discuss the thoughts, feelings, and solutions used.

When kids can see that adults also face challenges, that they also feel emotions like frustration, anger, and despair, as well as how diligence and perseverance help to overcome these feelings, they can begin to feel like they are also capable of taking on challenges.

Try to include your child in the problem-solving processes of your own challenges so that the two of you can try out their ideas.

Resilient children need to be allowed to take on age-appropriate difficult activities so that they can learn the value of discipline and focus. Determination requires kids to find and try out multiple solutions so that they can see what works for them.

Don't turn your child away when they come to you for help but also don't physically assist them. Rather, discuss what they are finding challenging specifically, and then let them unpack their solutions, using you as a sounding board. Once they have done that, you can watch and praise their effort as they implement their solutions.

2. Brainstorm As Much As Possible

Brainstorming allows your child to go through a set of solutions to a problem and helps them to weigh the outcomes of these solutions through trial and error. When your kid is about to quit, remove them from the task at hand, help them to calm down using the correct coping techniques, and then begin the brainstorming process.

Overcoming frustration this way ensures your child goes through the three-step calm down, brainstorm, and reflection process as a habit whenever they're faced with a new task or challenge in their life.

Adults need to take a backseat to young brainstormers so that they feel completely in control of the solutions and outcomes. When kids feel in control—that they are in the driver's seat—they are more invested in creating a solution, as well as more likely to take responsibility for the outcomes.

Resist the urge to help by offering solutions you see, and let your child develop their own sense of how to overcome their challenges.

3. Always Model the Right Behaviors

If you want your child to become gritty and resilient you need to model this behavior. That means you have to be emotionally intelligent, gritty, passionate, and empathetic in your own life too.

Trust me when I say, you can guide your child to be resilient and gritty all you want but if you are not emulating grittiness in your own behavior, they're simply going to follow your poor behavior.

Give your child real-life examples of how adversity is overcome when you don't quit, and celebrate with them when they overcome.

4. Give Your Children Examples Of Overcoming Failure

Adults have experienced failure far more than kids, and the fact that most of us still carry on with life proves that we have moved on from these failures. For kids to be resilient they need to understand that failure is a part of life and that when you accept it and move past it you can learn and grow.

Don't hide your failures from your children, and as long as the failure is age-appropriate, discuss these failures openly. Let your child know how you moved past these failures, and let them know how your life improved from the growth you experienced.

When you make a mistake in real-time, use it as a teachable moment so that your child can see that no one is perfect and that it's what you do with your mistakes and failures that count.

5. Remain Within the Bounds of Constructive Criticism

People need criticism in order to improve, and without constructive criticism, a person will never learn to reflect on what went right and what went wrong when facing issues. Parents need to see themselves as a support system or life coach to their child, and should never be harsh in their criticism.

But, for the message to truly come across, parents need to be open to constructive criticism and need to make sure that they are not harshly criticizing others. Model the behaviors of self-motivation and self-reflection, critiquing your own performance and ask your child for their feedback.

Use your words carefully, and make sure that you are sticking to the behaviors you expect from your child. The same applies to yourself, don't use words like 'stupid', or "too hard" when constructively criticizing yourself. Rather, highlight the challenge and then decide what went wrong with the process as well as what went right and then formulate the best way forward.

Passionate, Purposeful Kids

'Passion' and 'purpose' may be new buzzwords among the self-help community but successful people have always known that aside from grit and resilience, passion is the single most important driving force behind success.

Kids are naturally passionate about the things they love but parents need to be able to instill a passion for life with all that it is. Passion is the sum total of everything we are as a person and the motivation behind what we do. Not allowing your child to be passionate, or encouraging them to only be passionate in their strengths limits how diverse and interesting their life could be.

For children, passion needs to be tapped from their natural curiosity and their need to learn about everything the world has to offer. It ensures that their mindset is set to one that embraces growth and that they play to their strengths while working on their weaknesses.

How you choose to teach your child to live with purpose and passion is largely up to you, but there are some key points that need to be focused on.

In a world that is filled with harsh criticism and the expectation of perfection plastered all over television and the internet, it can be challenging to compassionately teach passion and drive. We want our children to know that it is great to go after what they want to achieve but that this should never be at the expense of others, and so we water down passion or we hope that by fueling our children's passion that they will instinctively know to consider others in the process.

But, once again, are we modeling the behavior we want to see in our children, or are we handing them a set of tools and expecting them to create a passionate life?

Kids are not much different from you when it comes to passion—they're passionate about what matters to them. And so it is important that you find out what it is that makes your child tick. For your child to be passionate about life and all of its challenges they need to be able to motivate themselves enough to push through the hard things with purpose.

Ultimately, purpose and passion go hand-in-hand, and in an education environment that does not value purpose, parents are charged almost solely with helping their children to ignite their passion.

Parents need to focus on not just teaching their kids skills but in fostering a sense of purpose while teaching, as well as equipping them with the correct emotional skills to deal with temptation, frustration, and self-doubt.

Remember that when a child doesn't know the reason behind what they are doing they are less likely to complete a task when it becomes challenging and that is why passion equals purpose which equates to success.

To foster passion in a child we first need to ascertain what their purpose is and no one really knows what their purpose is except the person themselves. Children need to feel comfortable enough to tell you what they believe their purpose is, and as parents, we need to be flexible enough to know that a purpose may change as a child grows and matures.

Find out what matters most to your child and you will know what is motivating their behaviors, and in turn, will know what their purpose is. Do they want to get good grades, be the best at a sport, want to create, dance, sing, educate? Whatever it is, your job is to decode their dreams and aspirations to a core purpose and then help your child to hone in and use that passion to achieve their goals.

It's important to understand that your child will probably not know what they want to do or be in the world, or how they would like to contribute until much later on. Actually, there are many adults out there who still aren't sure, and that's okay. As long as you are igniting passion, your child will focus on the task at hand because they will have a sense of purpose and this will drive them to keep going, even when things get tough.

Passion begins with you, and how you choose to foster it in your child. Never try to force your child to be passionate about something. Passion is not something that can be forced; it can only be inspired and motivated through encouragement, compassion, and inspiration.

Let's recap some of the skills and behaviors that will ignite passion in your child:

Nurture and teach emotional, empathy, and social skills. Empathetic children will pursue their passions with a purpose but will still keep others in mind as they move toward their goals.

Expose your kids to inspirational people who are their age and younger. Make sure to play your children inspirational and emotional videos and podcasts, let them read about other people's success journeys, and highlight the value of passion and purpose.

Listen to your children with the intention of hearing and understanding what they are saying to you. Don't make choices for your kids, and don't interrupt them when they come to you with their big ideas and dreams. Rather, ask your child how they will make their dreams come to fruition and never tell them that what they believe is impossible. Keep in mind that belief is subjective and what you believe is impossible, others will believe it is more than possible.

Expose your kids to a variety of interests and experiences and let them decide what they are passionate about. But, don't allow your child to be wishy-washy. Commitment is extremely important in life so make sure that when your child commits to a choice that they stick it out for a certain period of time before they move on to the next thing. Model a sense of purpose for your child and speak to them about the ups and downs, frustrations, and success in your life. Permit your child to see you as human and flawed so that they can see that perfection and passion are two very different things.

Guide them to their purpose, don't dictate to them what they should be purposeful in. Kids who are forced to follow activities they are not passionate about will become resentful and rebellious, ultimately following their passions later in life anyway.

Don't limit your kid's dreams, no matter how wildly ridiculous or fantastic they are, let your child dream. In fact, encourage them to dream, and to do it big! When a child is allowed to dream and to express their dreams they develop a sense that they have the ability to achieve these dreams. And a child's dreams will eventually become goals that they set. By encouraging your child to dream, and then brainstorming how to fulfill these dreams, you are teaching them how to set the milestones that will allow them to succeed at the goals they set later in life.

Yes, it is tough to stand aside as we watch our children struggle through life. Perhaps your child is the best reader in class, or your first grader draws and paints like a fifth-grader, but they will not try anything outside of their strengths. Maybe you find yourself justifying that they are working to their strengths, and because of that you never encourage them to try anything outside of their talents and strengths.

But in life, we need to be diversified, we need to be able to overcome challenges and we absolutely have to get up and dust ourselves off in order for us to succeed at anything.

It's frustrating and painful to see your child fall down, time and time again. It's even harder to see them experience disappointment and defeat, but you have to remind yourself that the most powerful tool for success is persistently pushing through mistakes.

It is important to remember that your child's frustration is just as painful for them as it is for you, but overcoming this pain ultimately instills the confidence they need to take on the next challenge. And when your child does overcome an obstacle it becomes a great teachable moment for future issues in which you can remind them about how capable they are when they put their minds to achieving something.

Kids truly need to grasp the concept that mistakes are not fatal, and that when they choose to try and try again they will eventually succeed. Some kids are just naturally more gritty than others but, as you can now see, there are so many ways to help your child become gritty.

Challenge your children, teach them skills, and model the right behavior. Learn to become a gritty parent, and promote perseverance above IQ, strengths, and the outcomes. Always remember that it's the process that counts, and parenting is a process too. Find what works for you and for your child so that you can learn and grow in grittiness.

Chapter 8:

Do You Have Grit?— Strategies to Become a Gritty Parent

"The trees don't grow into the sky. But these outer boundaries of where we will, eventually, stop improving are simply irrelevant for the vast majority of us."— Angela Duckworth

Kids may need grit to succeed in life but parents do too. Parenting is challenging and can be outright hard at times. It requires practice every single day to get it right, and if you were one of those kids who were never taught grit, it can sometimes feel like you want to check out.

But there is no window where you can hand in your parenting card, and sooner or later you will need to toughen up and learn to become gritty yourself.

By now you will know that grit is the passion and the perseverance required for you to achieve long-term, meaningful goals, and what could be more meaningful than raising children into adults who thrive in life?

You cannot rely on talent when it comes to parenting, it is a skill, and one you will need to learn. No amount of intelligence, charisma, or charm is going to help you navigate parenthood—you need grit!

Parenting, like life, is a marathon, one in which you place one foot in front of the other, even when it gets hard.

Here are some of the key strategies you will need for yourself to become a gritty parent and raise children with grit.

Set Goals and Make Them SMART

Specific, measurable, achievable, relevant, time-bound, (SMART) goals are necessary for people to achieve success in their life. Using SMART as a chosen method for setting goals ensures that your outcome, objectives, and actions required to achieve success are crystal clear. It ensures that smaller goals, or milestones, are achievable and realistically align with the end goal. Duckworth suggests using a method coined by Warren Buffet in which goals can be united.

Here's how:

- Write down 25 goals—Make sure they are realistic.

- Circle the five goals that are the highest priority for you.

- Take a look at the remaining goals and decide which of these are in line with your five priority goals.

- Eliminate any goals that will have you working against your top five goals.

- Now employ SMART and set your milestones.

Finally, pursue your milestones. Goals that are not pursued are merely dreams that will never be achieved.

Rediscover Your Passion

Adults tend to set aside their passions to fulfill the needs of others. Whether these people are their employers, their spouse, friends, or even their kids, is irrelevant. When you give up your passion, you begin to work without a purpose, and this is a dangerous state of being, especially when you're trying to raise gritty kids.

It is important that you find interests outside of your job or your professional life, and that you not only dedicate time and effort to these interests but see which of them ignites passion in your life once more. You need to set time aside for yourself to rediscover what you like, how you think, and what it is that you truly care about outside of your family and work.

Once you have identified these, make sure to:

- Attend, practice, and participate deliberately in your activities. Don't make excuses that others need your time more.

- Set a personal goal that accommodates this passion.

- Make sure to eliminate distractions from your activities—multitasking is a myth.

- Reflect on your progress and be honest about what you want to achieve.

- Refine your process, always.

Reflect on Your Purpose

Once you have reignited your passion, it is time for you to reflect upon your purpose. Is your purpose to connect with others? To inspire those around you? To be innovative or creative?

Whatever you reaffirm your purpose to be, decide how your purpose fits with your goals and find ways to connect your goals and passions to your purpose. Your purpose will always be the deepest reflection of the values you hold onto. And once you reconnect with your purpose you will begin to work with passion and resilience, despite any obstacles that may be placed in your path.

Stop the Negative Self-Talk

Parents spend a whole lot of time criticizing their own actions and decisions, and often this is done in the harshest of ways. You simply cannot inspire yourself and others if you are constantly pulling yourself apart for the things you say and do.

When you find yourself criticizing yourself it is important to stop and ask yourself one question, *"Would I say this to the people I love and value the most?"* If your answer is no then it is time to reframe your internal conversations and begin to institute constructive criticism in your life. No one is perfect, and we're all going to make mistakes in life, it's what you choose to do with those mistakes that counts.

Surround Yourself With the Right People

We expect our kids to drown out negative people and those who are a bad influence on their behaviors or their mental health, yet as adults, we tend to drag around dead weight because of some sense of responsibility or loyalty.

Unfortunately, negative people need to reach their own turning point to positivity, and some will never do that because they lack the grit and determination to work through the difficult processes needed for a positive mindset.

Now I'm not recommending you cut people out of your life because sometimes this just isn't possible, but you can choose to limit your time with these people, or change your own mindset to one of acceptance of their behaviors and resolve to not allow it affect you.

With all of this in mind, it is important to acknowledge that some people are just not worth our time or our mental health, and if you identify these kinds of people in your life it may be time to move on.

SMART Goal Setting for Parents

Setting SMART goals for your career and personal achievements will set you up for success in those fields but have you ever thought about what your goals are as a parent?

Take a look at this list and see which of these sound familiar:

- I will not lose my patience.
- My kids will only have healthy snack alternatives.
- My kids will spend less time online and more time experiencing life.

- I will put down my phone and pay attention when my child talks to me.

Chances are that you have tried to commit to at least one of the items on this endless list. But what happens when your kid comes running past you, Xbox controller in one hand, mouth full of Cheetos while they gleefully try to catch the dog who probably has something important clenched between his teeth—all the while you are on an important client call that during which you asked your children to please remain under control for 15 minutes?

It's likely your goals will go flying out the window in a moment. Despondent, you ask yourself why you just cannot seem to set parenting goals, stick to them, and achieve one of them for even the shortest period of time.

The truth is that the goals listed above are only going to set you up for failure because they're, a) not really realistic, and b) you're dealing with a pretty changeable, chaotic external factor, that being your child.

So how do you set realistic SMART goals as a parent? How do you turn inward instead of handing part of the responsibility of achieving your goals to a tiny person who is still learning the right way to behave and how to self-regulate?

Decide What You Want to Achieve as a Parent

Because SMART goals require the goal to be achievable and realistic, it is important to step outside of the box when deciding what you want to achieve. Unlike career and personal goals, your parenting goals include another person or people who have their own objectives and goals.

When you create your parenting goals ask yourself:

- What memories would you like to experience with your kid?

- What are your relationship goals for your child?

- How would you like to inspire your child?

- What common interests would you like to develop?

- What values and beliefs would you like to instill?

Setting goals as a parent is more about helping you to build a meaningful relationship with your child so that they mimic the behavior that you model for them while you achieve your personal and career goals.

Your parenting goals should never be about what you want your child to become, that is their responsibility.

Instead, you should set goals that help you to become the parent you want to be for your child.

These goals should include how you will develop grit in your child, focusing on their strengths and weaknesses, and providing them with the skills they need to become successful.

Ultimately, the decision to become gritty and successful will lay with your child when they are older and I promise you that your child is not going to remember that you had to take an important call while they were playing. They are going to remember what you did with them, what values you instilled in them, the skills you equipped them with, and how you chose to create great memories.

Setting Those Goals

As a parent, you will need to surrender to the chaos of living with kids, and sometimes, some of the best memories made will come from those moments.

Breaking down the SMART goal-setting process will make it easier for you to identify, institute, and pursue the goals you have as a parent.

- **SPECIFIC–**Your goals need to be specific to what you want to achieve. "I want to succeed in creating an open relationship with my child." For younger children, you can make these goals skills-based, "I will teach my child how to get dressed in the morning without assistance by the end of next month."

- **MEASURABLE–**The results of the goal must be measurable to avoid the goal and its milestones being vague. "I will spend more time with my child," should be replaced with, "I will dedicate 30 minutes every day to an activity with my child, preferably an activity they would like to do."

- **ACTIONABLE–**A goal or milestone not pursued is useless. It is important to pursue your milestones in order to achieve your goals. Actionable goals are tough because we sometimes frame them in a way that sets us up for failure. So, instead of saying, "I promise not to lose my temper with my kids," say, "When I feel like my patience is wearing thin I will remove myself from the situation and count to 10."

- **REALISTIC–**Goals need to be realistic so that you are not fighting against an already hectic life. This is the difference between, "I will only feed my child healthy food," and, "I will offer my child healthy choices so that they can learn to eat healthily."

- **TIME-BOUND–**You need to set a realistic timeframe for you to achieve your goals. Some goals will be long-term, while others will be short-term. Whatever the time may be, make sure that you are setting a time frame to achieve your goal. An example of this is, "I will teach my child how to prepare their own packed lunch for the next 30 days. After day 31, my child will pack their own lunch from the choices I give them."

Your goals should be written down along with the increments or milestones required to achieve these goals. Remember that parenting goals are not going to be easy. You are, after all, setting goals that involve other people. It is important to act on your milestones, and celebrate when you achieve these milestones.

Review and Reflect

Finally, remember that life happens and that sometimes your milestones will need to be tweaked to fit in with your child's schedule and with yours. Changing milestones is not a reason to move the goalposts or abandon your goals, but when plan a isn't working it only makes sense to move to plan b.

To effectively manage your milestones, and to have them remain relevant, you will need to take some time to review and reflect upon what is working and what is not.

Reviewing and reflecting on where you stand with your goals should be done by turning inward and seeing how well you are implementing the steps required to achieve your goals. But, it is important that you also ask the people affected by your goals how you and they are doing.

Ask your child how they believe you are doing, be open and honest about your objectives, and let your child help you brainstorm any changes that may need to be made. Take time to reflect upon how your child's behaviors have changed; are they progressing, do they enjoy working toward your goals with you, how are you feeling about your child's progress?

Reviewing and reflecting upon your goals and progress is a critical part of successfully achieving what you have set out to do.

Strengthening Your Relationship With Your Kid

For your child, the relationship you choose to build with them will be the most important connection of their life. Your words and actions have a profound effect on your child and how they view the world, and a parent-child relationship that is strong, and positive will ensure that you and your child can take on all of the challenges that come your way throughout your lives.

Having a strong relationship with your child begins and ends with spending quality time with them in which you choose to foster your bond with them. And because every child is different, you will need to find out what works for you when you are spending time with your kid.

Perhaps you don't know where to start when strengthening your relationship or you may just be looking for a way to solidify your relationship, and when it comes to a child-parent relationship, there is no such thing as a relationship that is too strong.

Say I Love You, But Show it Too

People have different love languages and it's important that you ascertain what your child's love language is, but regardless of whether they are words of affirmation, or action-orientated, it's important to show that you love them as much as you tell them. Find out how your child perceives love and then practice these forms with them. Make sure to express your love through eye contact, open and honest conversations, dedicated time, and expressions of love like hugs.

Tell Your Child You Love Them

Your child may tell you that they don't want to hear the words I love you often but they do need to hear them, and they should be said by you with honesty and with purpose at least once every single day. Saying I love you reaffirms that your feelings for them are unconditional and unequivocal and that regardless of their behavior, your love is unshakable. Saying I love you, especially when your child is having a bad day, or is particularly unruly, will let them know that you are capable of separating behavior from the person whom you love.

Be Unshakable Regarding Consequences of Breaking Rules

Kids need structure to thrive, learn and grow in the world. Your child needs to know what you expect of them, what behaviors are acceptable, and what the consequences are for their behaviors. Kids need to earn privileges and need to know that they are free to explore the world around them within the boundaries you set for them. Rules should be age-appropriate to allow kids to experience and take on more responsibility.

The same applies to the consequences of stepping outside of the boundaries set for them—consequences need to be age-appropriate. Above everything rules and boundaries need to be consistently enforced so that your child knows that they cannot manipulate their way out of trouble.

Empathize With Your Child

You will never know how to parent, guide, and inspire your child to greatness if you don't take the time to listen to what they have to say and empathize with them. It is important that you acknowledge and validate their feelings, showing them that you are, at the very least, trying to understand the world from your child's point of view.

Seeking to hear and understand your child will help to build mutual respect and will ensure that your child is comfortable coming to you with issues they are facing.

Play With Your Child Often

Kids learn the skills they will need in the adult world through play and as such, it is important that you spend time playing with your child. Kids learn everything from language to emotions, creativity, and relationship-building skills through playing with other kids and with the adults in their lives.

Enjoy time with your child during which you enrich and play with them so that they can not only learn the skills they need to thrive but also understand that you are committed to spending one on one time with them.

Set Aside Uninterrupted Time

When setting aside one-on-one quality time to play with your child, make sure that this time is uninterrupted. Do not set yourself up to spend time with them when you know you are within business hours or when you will need to check in on emails or technology. Your focus needs to be solely on your child when you are with them.

Let your child know that you are committed to them, and that you value the time you spend with them. Explain to them that you will only check your phone to make sure it is not an emergency and then stick with that.

In the grander scheme of things, not answering an email, or not answering a call for 30 minutes is really not going to make much difference, but if you cannot commit to not being 100% in the moment, schedule your daily one-on-one time so that it will be uninterrupted.

Eat Together

One of the biggest issues families face today is a disconnect because they have moved away from the dining table to the television. Sitting together to eat at least one meal a day is an invaluable, interruption-free time in which families can reconnect and share what has happened during their day.

Everyone, including you, should put their devices away and focus on conversations about the day. Added to this, eating together is a great teachable moment in which you can encourage healthy eating habits, and mindful practices.

Use your mealtimes with your kids to impart knowledge and teach them valuable skills by first listening to what they are telling you, and then guiding them into conversations that will benefit them.

Put Rituals into Place With Your Children

Make sure that you have rituals in place, and if you have more than one kid, make sure that these rituals include one-on-one time with each child as an individual. Your children do need to know that they are part of a greater unit, but they also need to know that they are valued and worthy of time alone with their parents. These rituals can be monthly 'dates' or activities that allow you to observe and reward or celebrate your child for the unique person they are and the successes they have achieved.

Look for the Good

Some kids are difficult. They act out for various reasons and when a child is in a difficult phase it can be very hard to praise good behaviors because they're so few and far between. Your job as a parent is to find these good moments and really affirm the great behavior. The point is not to look past bad behaviors but to find the minutes of good, and let your child know that you are proud of them for trying to get through what is going on in their life right now.

Resisting the Urge to Competitively Parent

If you've ever gone to a PTA meeting or a sports event at your kid's school, you will have noticed that there are always 'those' parents who are talking about everything their child has achieved or accomplished in their day.

And, if you're like me, these conversations can have you worrying about what your children are doing, or not doing, or if you're being the best parent you can possibly be.

If you're a parent reading this book, chances are that you really care about whether or not you're raising your child right. It's only natural to love and adore your kids and to want to invest in their future; you could even say that you're passionate about it!

But all of this leads to a bit of a conundrum and a huge temptation to become one of 'those' parents who are constantly trying to outdo the next. You listen in on their conversations, nervously wondering if you are on track with parenting and if your child is progressing well as they mature.

It's not easy being a modern parent. There are so many definitions of what good parenting is, and what kids need, and we, as parents, seem to have lost the simplicity of being a good parent. And yes, modern kids have a whole host of new temptations and traps they can fall into because life is not quite as simple, but parenting only needs to be complicated if you make it so.

Which brings me back to competitive parenting—a world in which a child, and by default their parent, can only be deemed successful if the kid excels at everything from academics, to cultural, creative, spiritual, and social activities. We are so caught up in what 'those' parents will say about our sometimes messy, sometimes chaotic child that we lose the value of what it means to be a parent.

This conscious creation of kids into Stepford'ish human beings inadvertently leads to competition, not just in the parents but in the children, and this competition is not the healthy kind. In fact, those obnoxious, bragard parents generally will produce children who appear to be outwardly confident, but who are living with anxiety, feelings of inadequacy, and a sense of self-criticism that is extremely unhealthy.

Competitive parenting is not healthy, not for you, and not for your child. You are not nurturing or fostering success, but controlling your child and breaking their spirit in the hopes that you will be the best parent.

Control, in itself, is damaging as it tells your child that you have no belief in them or their ability to make good choices in their own lives. At its very best, competitive parenting places a child under pressure they're not meant to deal with, and at its worst, a child will feel that they are only a good person if they do, say, and achieve what their parents expect of them.

Because of this, it is vitally important that you resist the urge to hop into the "my child does or has achieved this circle." And when you feel the draw of being a perfect parent to a perfect child, remember that your child is so incredibly unique. They are only created by you on a biological and cellular level, and while you can guide them, inspire them, and motivate them, you cannot truly create them because they will become the sum total of the choices, relationships, and experiences they have had in their life.

If you are forcing these choices on your child, all you are doing is snuffing out their light, and, ironically, dooming their future success.

The perfect parent doesn't exist. It is a fallacy. Your only job is to equip your children with the skills they need to become successful, to offer them good choices, and to instill great values like determination and grit so that when they move on to adulthood, they can look back and say my parents were great because they taught me how to thrive in life.

Conclusion

"Whatever their parents' education or income, all children really need the same thing: appropriately demanding challenges in combination with consistently warm and respectful support."— Angela Duckworth

Modern parenting is filled with uncertainty and so many questions. "How do I raise my child to be successful, compassionate, and kind, but resilient?"

The good news is that modern parents are not alone, and with the guidance of parents who learned along the way to get it right, gritty, resilient children can be created. Parents themselves need to learn how to be resilient though, especially if they have become caught up in their own fears on how to parent.

The first step in raising resilient children is to step away from the concept that children need to be wrapped in bubble wrap for them to be happy and healthy. We believe that these qualities will lead to them becoming successful and yes, that may be true, but success also requires all of the traits that make up grit.

Grit is not something that can be demanded, and kids will need to be inspired to greatness. You simply cannot dictate that they will be successful. It's important to nurture, inspire, guide, and reinforce the lessons we teach them so that they can become the successful adults we hope they will become.

While time spent considering parenting strategies is great, parents and educators need to implement what they have learned so that kids can go out into the world able to apply what they have learned.

When children are infants and toddlers, their grit is exceptional. Through sheer determination, kids will learn to do everything from sitting up to walking, talking, dressing themselves, etc. When our kids are babies, we praise and encourage their gritty behavior, celebrating each milestone achieved. But once your child enters into the next phase of their life, you intervene, terrified that the one thing that taught them the essential skills to grow and develop will lead them to harm.

I'm not saying you should not protect your child from absolute harm, but some pain, frustration, and discomfort are all part of the learning process. Parents forget that their actions contribute more to your child's determination being chipped away than the pain and discomfort they feel.

Now is the time to stop interrupting your frustrated child and allow them to complete the task that is frustrating them. Because grit is the only way your child will learn how to push through life's challenges and obstacles. Kids need to know that they hold the power to overcome issues and have the ability to achieve their life's goals.

While grit is great, it is important to incorporate a growth mindset in your child as well. These two concepts may go hand-in-hand but they are distinctively different and you can, technically, have a growth mindset without grit. You simply cannot, however, have grit without a growth mindset.

Kids who are raised with a growth mindset may develop grit as a natural byproduct but grit requires a person to become tenacious in life. Gritty people know that goals are not meant to be moved around and that long-term goals and dreams need to be consistently pursued. When kids are developed to be gritty, they learn to work smarter and harder so that they can succeed. Grit when coupled with a growth mindset creates a child that is unstoppable in the pursuit of their goals while still working within their morals, principles, and values.

Part of being gritty is to have passion because passion is the driving force and the desire to achieve anything they set their mind to. Passion is less about the outcome and more about the process to become successful.

People who live a life without passion are rudderless and will not find their purpose, or may only find their purpose much later in life. For your child to live a life in which their infinite dreams are achievable they will need to live their life with passion and purpose. Inspiring your child to nurture their dreams and to convert those dreams into achievable goals is one of the greatest gifts you will give them because courageous, passionate kids are the ones who are happy, balanced, and driven to succeed.

Children need courage and for your child to grow and develop in life they will need to be able to set their fear aside. Courage helps your child do the right thing even when others are doing the wrong thing and it ensures that your kid will admit to their mistakes when they make them. Without courage, it will be extremely difficult for any kid to persevere through life's goals and challenges. For your child to develop a healthy self-esteem they will need to have the courage to try new things and persevere through the tough bits.

And, perseverance is not a characteristic kids are short of if you allow them to tap into their tenacity and their natural instincts to learn. Where adults apply perseverance to mental hurdles, the reality is that perseverance should encompass anything and everything that is difficult to overcome. For children, these could be obstacles like learning a new physical skill, forming new habits, education, creative skills like arts and dance, and even social and relationship skills. Kids need to be allowed to figure out how they can push through these obstacles.

Children don't understand the limitations we place on them until they're older and they believe that they aren't capable because we have shown them it is easier for Mom and Dad to complete the tasks for them. It is vitally important for you to instill perseverance so that your kid can conscientiously work toward their goals.

Conscientious kids will perform tasks and approach life with a thorough, vigilant approach. When children are taught how to be conscientious they develop the ability to overcome their frustrations and tackle the task at hand with patience and to the best of their ability. It instills the innate ability to identify that a task done well the first time around saves time and more hard work. Teach your child to work conscientiously so that they can be more organized and only have to complete a task once. Show them the value of working smart, hard, and properly while tapping into their curiosity so that your child wastes less time, and knows how to methodically take tasks on.

Allow your child to be curious, and encourage them to approach new tasks with an open mind so that they can work through each new task with diligence and a can-do attitude. When your child learns to embrace anything new with a methodical, conscientious approach, they begin to understand that every task ticked off the list will be done to the best of their ability.

Always remember that kids have a built-in ability to work through the many challenges they face in life. Children who are equipped well can cope with the normal, age-appropriate stresses and strains of life without intervention and when parents try to shield their children from these normal obstacles they remove their children's confidence. A child who isn't confident finds it difficult to overcome problems and their ability to bounce back from failures and adversity becomes much harder. Kids need to be resilient if they are to cope in a tough adult world.

Teach your child to be courageous, curious, and passionate about the world around them, allow them to be resilient, and show them how they can come back from mistakes and failure. Because ultimately children need to be allowed to be brave, curious and trusting of their natural instincts. Trust your child to make the right decisions but remain close to help them when it is absolutely necessary. Allow them to step safely outside of their comfort zone and praise them for their efforts. Let your child push the limits of life so that they can learn, grow, and become resilient, gritty people who succeed in life.

References

Bergold, S., & Steinmayr, R. (2018). Personality and Intelligence Interact in the Prediction of Academic Achievement. *Journal of Intelligence*, *6*(2), 27. https://doi.org/10.3390/jintelligence6020027

Duckworth, A. (2015). *Angela Duckworth*. Angela Duckworth. https://angeladuckworth.com/research/

Duckworth, A., & Gross, J. J. (2014). Self-Control and Grit. *Current Directions in Psychological Science*, *23*(5), 319–325. https://doi.org/10.1177/0963721414541462

Dweck, C. S., Butterfield, B., Lamb, J., Good, C., & Mangels, J. A. (2006). Why do beliefs about intelligence influence learning success? A social cognitive neuroscience model. *Social Cognitive and Affective Neuroscience*, *1*(2), 75–86. https://doi.org/10.1093/scan/nsl013

Ginsburg, K. R., & Carlson, E. C. (2011). Resilience in action: an evidence-informed, theoretically driven approach to building strengths in an office-based setting. *Adolescent Medicine: State of* the Art Reviews, *22*(3), 458–481, xi. https://pubmed.ncbi.nlm.nih.gov/22423460/

Grit Quotes by Angela Duckworth. (2016). Goodreads.com. https://www.goodreads.com/work/quotes/45670634-grit-passion-perseverance-and-the-science-of-success

Jarrett, C. (2018). *How our teenage years shape our personalities.* Bbc.com; BBC Future. https://www.bbc.com/future/article/20180608-how-our-teenage-years-shape-our-personalities

Matthews, T., Fisher, H. L., Bryan, B. T., Danese, A., Moffitt, T. E., Qualter, P., Verity, L., & Arseneault, L. (2021). This is what loneliness looks like: A mixed-methods study of loneliness in adolescence and young adulthood. *International Journal of Behavioral Development*, 016502542097935. https://doi.org/10.1177/0165025420979357

Shi, B., Cao, X., Chen, Q., Zhuang, K., & Qiu, J. (2017). Different brain structures associated with artistic and scientific creativity: a voxel-based morphometry study. *Scientific Reports, 7*(1). https://doi.org/10.1038/srep42911

www.ingramcontent.com/pod-product-compliance
Lightning Source LLC
Chambersburg PA
CBHW030302100526
44590CB00012B/485